# How safe is your baby...?

The facts behind the official advice

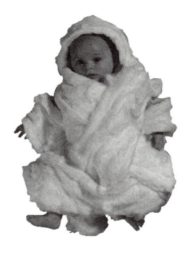

## Annie Vickerstaff

**Editors Richard Craze, Roni Jay**

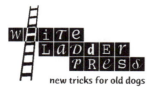
WHiTe LaDdEr PRESS
new tricks for old dogs

Published by White Ladder Press Ltd
Great Ambrook, Near Ipplepen, Devon TQ12 5UL
01803 813343
www.whiteladderpress.com

First published in Great Britain in 2006

10 9 8 7 6 5 4 3 2 1

© Annie Vickerstaff 2006

The right of Annie Vickerstaff to be identified as author of this work has been asserted by her in accordance with the Copyright, Designs and Patents Act 1988.

10-digit ISBN 1 905410 06 9
13-digit ISBN 978 1 905410 06 4

British Library Cataloguing in Publication Data
A CIP record for this book can be obtained from the British Library.

Design and typesetting by Martin Bristow

Cover design by Sarah Davies

Cover photograph by Imagestate

Printed and bound by TJ International Ltd, Padstow, Cornwall

Cover printed by St Austell Printing Company, St Austell, Cornwall

Printed on totally chlorine-free paper

| WORCESTERSHIRE COUNTY COUNCIL | | |
|---|---|---|
| | 491 | |
| Bertrams | | 12.11.06 |
| 618.24 | | £7.99 |
| WY | | |

**White Ladder Press Ltd**
**Great Ambrook, Near Ipplepen, Devon TQ12 5UL**
**01803 813343**
**www.whiteladderpress.com**

VICKERSTAFF, A.          618.24

How safe is your baby?: the facts
behind the official advice

70002986491          Pbk

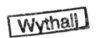

Please return/renew this item by the last date shown

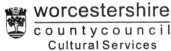

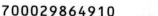

Cultural Services

# Contents

## Dedication

This is for my mum, Gloria, who wanted a nice little girl but ended up with me instead. Thanks for not minding, mum – love you xxx.

## Acknowledgements

Many thanks to midwife and health visitor Carolyn Westwood for reading the manuscript and passing on her professional advice and comments.

## Disclaimer

*How Safe is Your Baby* is intended as a resource, providing accurate and unbiased information so that you as parents can make up your own minds as to risks and benefits. It is not intended to replace medical advice and should not be read as such. Much effort has gone into sourcing accurate, solid, good quality scientific research wherever possible, but time flies like an arrow (and fruit flies like a banana): things change and information can become outdated. Neither the author, nor the publisher, can be held liable or responsible for any loss or claim arising out of the use or misuse of this book or the information it provides. Your decisions are entirely your own, and it is our purpose to empower you in your choices but not to persuade you one way or the other.

# Introduction

As someone once said, if you suggest that a chicken and a horse have something in common because they have an average of 3 legs each, you're statistically correct but factually barking. Lots of stats are like this, and you can go through life perfectly happily not knowing any of them. However, there's a lot of really scary stuff out there about the health and safety of your baby, all backed up by imposing sets of figures, and unfortunately we have to deal with the stats in order to find a balance.

So what's this book about? You may be anxious about the safety of the MMR vaccine, you may be unsure whether you can eat cheese while pregnant, you might be worried you'll catch toxoplasmosis and pass it on to your baby – there's a minefield of information out there that's confusing, concerning or just downright contradictory, and as a busy parent (or parent-to-be) you just don't have time to trawl through reams of data to find the truth. Well, don't worry: I've done it for you.

There's a lot of medical research in this book, but I've put it neatly at the end of each section so it doesn't slow you down. It's all referenced so you can check it, and it's from sound, reliable authorities wherever possible. The aim here is to give you the official line and the alternatives, so you can decide what you want to do.

It's my hope that, once you've read this book, you'll ignore most of it and go on about your business of having a happy, healthy baby who will ruin your sleep, be sick all over your furniture and produce weapons-grade poo, just like any other normal infant.

# Part 1

# Pregnancy

## 1 Folic acid

When it occurs naturally in foods, folic acid is known as folate. It is one of the family of B vitamins (B9). It's a vital ingredient of spinal fluid, and if you don't have enough of it in your body, there is a risk of your baby having neural tube defects. This is when the tube that surrounds and protects the central nervous system doesn't completely close up. The most common neural tube defect is spina bifida.

### Spina bifida

Spina bifida means 'split spine'. The backbone usually provides a protective tube of bones with the nerves (spinal cord) running down the middle. In spina bifida, the bones do not close round the spinal cord and the nerves can bulge out on the unborn baby's back and become damaged. This happens very early on in the first 4 weeks of pregnancy. One in every 1,500 babies in the UK is affected. Folic acid has been shown to reduce the risk of neural tube defects in the developing foetus.

If you're intending to become pregnant, current medical advice is to take 400mcgs (micrograms) of folic acid daily from the time you stop using contraception, continuing this for the first 3 months of pregnancy. Below is a list of foods that either contain folate, or are fortified with it, so will help to give you the folate you need naturally (around 300mcgs of dietary folate a day ideally). If you do decide to take a supplement, remember to consider the advice to ensure that vitamin A or fish liver oil are not included, as there is a limit to how much vitamin A you're supposed to have while pregnant.

- fortified breads and cereals
- papaya
- oranges
- brown rice
- spinach
- kale
- broccoli
- cabbage
- parsnips
- iceberg lettuce
- black eyed beans
- the good old Brussels sprout

You're advised to eat your veg raw or al dente as folate is reduced during cooking. The safety of folic acid was evaluated by the independent Expert Group on Vitamins and Minerals (EVM), which concluded that supplements of up to 1000mcg (1mg) daily is unlikely to do anyone any harm. Some women who are at high risk of having a baby affected by neural tube defect may be advised by their doctor to take over 1mg (milligram) of folic acid daily.

## Useful websites/references

**http://www.asbah.org/**
Association for Spina Bifida and Hydrocephalus

**http://www.eatwell.gov.uk/**
Food and nutrition

**http://www.shef.ac.uk/pregnancy_nutrition/index.php**
University of Sheffield Centre of Pregnancy Nutrition

**http://ods.od.nih.gov**
National Institutes of Health: Office of Dietary Supplements

# 2 What you can and can't eat

You can eat what you like: roast beef and custard, haddock ice cream, curried strawberries, whatever you fancy. There are risks with certain foods, such as soft, unpasteurised cheeses that may contain listeria, and below I've covered the most common sources of possible problems and what the risks are.

## Listeria

Listeriosis, caused by the bacterium listeria monocytogenes, is a rare infection affecting only 1-3 cases per million of the population per year, and around 1 in 30,000 live and stillbirths in England & Wales (estimate by the Chief Medical Officer). Listeria occurs naturally in soil and water, from where farm animals can pick it up. Although the animal itself may show no symptoms, its meat or milk can contain the bacterium and this can find its way into food and dairy products. Via manure, listeria can also affect vegetables, particularly root crops like potatoes and carrots. However, it's no good vowing to eat out of tins and packets, because processed foods can contain it too. Although pasteurisation and cooking destroy listeria, food can be reinfected after processing and before packaging.

### Symptoms and sources

Listeriosis resembles mild flu in pregnant women, but is able to cross the placenta, and can cause severe illness in a newborn baby (fortunately you can't transmit it via breast milk). It can also trigger miscarriage. Mould ripened soft cheeses (ie camembert and brie) are a common source of listeria, but it is also found in feta, blue veined cheeses, patés (including vegetarian), pre-washed salads, ready cooked poultry and cooked-chilled meals. Official advice is for pregnant mums to avoid listeria, as their immune systems are affected by hormonal changes and therefore less effective than usual. In fact this makes you 20 times more likely to succumb to listeriosis.

What about hard cheeses such as cheddar? Listeria is present in these, but at very low levels: less than 1 bacterium per gram. This is not considered to be a risk during pregnancy. If you fancy comforting yourself with a soft-whip ice cream from the nearest van, be aware that listeria can survive at surprisingly low temperatures, down to 0°C. This is a good reason for clearing out your fridge and disinfecting it (or getting your mother to do it).

## Salmonellosis

There are around 200 varieties of salmonella, and the effect they have on you can vary according to which one you've got. The most common ones for humans are: salmonellas typhi, typhimurium, enteritidis, and cholerasuis. As their names suggest, they will give you typhoid, enteritis and cholera, which are not nice at all. Salmonellosis is a common cause of food poisoning, often associated with raw poultry or meat and raw or lightly cooked eggs. It's been estimated that one in every 450 eggs may be contaminated with salmonella bacteria. Thorough cooking kills it, so the advice is to make sure both the yolk and the white of your egg is solid, and to avoid home made sorbets, meringues, mousses and mayonnaise, as these are often made with raw eggs. Mayo shop-bought in jars is considered fine, as it's made with pasteurised egg.

Cooking guidelines (medium sized eggs):
- Boil for at least 7 minutes or until indestructible
- Fry on both sides
- Poach for at least 5 minutes till the white is completely set and the yolk is firm.

It's possible that the outside of an egg can carry bacteria (it's been up a chicken's bum, remember) so to be sure of avoiding infection you need to keep eggs separate from other foods and wash your hands after handling them. Don't wash an egg: the shell is porous and can let contamination through into the contents.

Antacids can affect the ph of your stomach and make you more vulnerable to salmonella type infections. As your stomach acid is weaker during pregnancy anyway, you may well be more susceptible to orally contracted infections. Gastroenteritis is the most common manifestation of salmonella infection, causing nausea and vomiting, and often progressing to abdominal cramping and diarrhoea. The usual treatment is antibiotics, though the jury's out on whether these really do any good.

## Vitamin A

There has been some concern that high doses of this vitamin can cause birth defects, but opinions differ as to how significant the risk really is. The recommended daily allowance for vitamin A is 4000-8000 ius (international units). A 3 ounce serving of liver provides 30,000 ius. Beta carotene, found in fruit and veggies, is safe for pregnant women to take, and in fact most vitamin companies have switched to this form of vitamin A. The official advice is that Retinol, or preformed vitamin A, should be avoided in high doses just before conception and during the first weeks of pregnancy, ie not more than 3,300 mcg (micrograms) daily, so it's recommended that you avoid eating liver during this time. This includes fish liver oils, but not fish oils (these are extracted from the body of the fish) which are fine.

## Iron

Of course, liver is also one of the best sources of iron, helping to protect against anaemia (which is relatively common during pregnancy), so you'll have to make your own decision on whether to avoid liver altogether or to eat it, probably in moderation, depending on your view of the risk and your susceptibility to anaemia. The daily recommended allowance (RDA) for iron is 15mg, but as most of us don't manage to eat that much, when you become pregnant and need a bit extra you may not have the necessary reserves. Green leafy veg is iron-rich, and also wholemeal bread, fortified cereals, potatoes, lean red meat, shellfish, raisins, prunes and pulses. Vitamin C aids iron absorption, so orange juice and fresh fruit can help; you need to take them at the same time as the iron-rich food.

## Wacky stuff

There is some scientific evidence to suggest that if you use essential oils of clove and cinnamon atmospherically in an oil burner, this can inhibit the growth of listeria and staphyllococcus aurea, as well as yeasts (candida albicans) and moulds. But don't tell anyone I told you. **(1)**

## Useful websites/references

**http://www.cdc.gov**
Centers for Disease Control and Prevention (US site)

**www.babycentre.co.uk**
Fantastic, comprehensive website that's scientific, informative and friendly

**www.marchofdimes.com**
Great US parenting site

**http://www.shef.ac.uk/pregnancy_nutrition/index.php** University of Sheffield Centre of Pregnancy Nutrition

**http://ods.od.nih.gov**
National Institutes of Health: Office of Dietary Supplements

**http://www.amm.co.uk**
Association of Medical Microbiologists

**http://www.emedicine.com**
US professional medical site

**http://www.patient.co.uk**
UK patient health information

## Other references

1  Solid- and vapor-phase antimicrobial activities of six essential oils: susceptibility of selected foodborne bacterial and fungal strains.
Lopez P, Sanchez C, Batlle R, Nerin C.
Department of Analytical Chemistry, Aragon Institute of Engineering Research, CPS-University of Zaragoza, Maria de Luna st. 3, E-50018 Zaragoza, Spain.

# 3 Smoking

There are more that 2,500 chemicals in cigarette smoke. It's not known for sure which of these is harmful to a growing foetus, but both nicotine and carbon monoxide are believed to be damaging.

Women who smoke have an increased risk of about 40% of delaying conception by over a year. Smoking almost doubles a woman's chances of having a low birthweight baby, and this is one of the leading causes of infant illness, including premature birth, the possibility of lifelong disabilities like cerebral palsy, mental under development and learning problems, or even foetal death. 12.2% of babies born to smoking mothers in the USA in 2002 weighed less than $5^1/_2$ lb at birth, compared with 7.5% of those born to non-smoking mums.

## SIDS

Babies whose mothers smoke during pregnancy are up to 3 times more likely die from Sudden Infant Death Syndrome (SIDS). Smoking also increases the risk of complications during pregnancy. It can double the risk of placental problems, ie placenta praevia and placental abruption, and can increase the risk of premature rupture of the membranes, leading to premature birth.

## Cleft lip or palate

One study showed that mothers who smoked 20 or more cigarettes a day were doubling their baby's chances of being born with a cleft lip or cleft palate. This risk increases to 8 times if there is also a genetic predisposition.

## ADD

Children born to smoking mothers have a higher incidence of hyperactivity and Attention Deficit Disorder. Their brains may be smaller and less developed, they may have a lower IQ and a higher risk of learning problems.

In the 40s and 50s, textbooks rarely mentioned hyperactivity in school age children – it just wasn't a very common problem. Today it's estimated that between 5% and 10% of children in the USA have some sort of hyperactive behavioural problem or Attention Deficit Disorder (1). Studies note that the rise of such problems in children coincides with the wide expansion of cigarette smoking among the adult population, particularly in women. According to an article in Neurotoxicology and Teratology it has been found that the children of smoking mothers have auditory processing difficulties, meaning it is more difficult for them to focus on what a teacher is saying, to follow directions, or to remember what the teacher has said. (2)

An article in Archives of General Psychiatry concludes that:

"Maternal smoking during pregnancy appears to be a robust independent risk factor for conduct disorder in male offspring. Maternal smoking during pregnancy may have direct adverse effects on the developing foetus or be a marker for a [so far] unmeasured characteristic of mothers that is of etiologic significance for conduct disorder." (Etiologic significance= a causative factor) (3)

Babies of smokers can show signs of withdrawal similar to those manifested by babies of drug addicts, and can be more jittery and difficult to calm. And all these problems still apply even if you're not a smoker, but you are constantly exposed to the second hand smoke of others.

## Smoking after the birth

Exposing your baby to smoke after it's born can give it a higher risk of lower respiratory tract diseases such as bronchitis and pneumonia, and also ear problems, ie glue ear and middle ear infections. Not to mention an increased risk of meningitis. Your baby will passively smoke the equivalent of 60-150 cigarettes a year. Exposure in early years can lead to asthma. A toddler who lives with a parent who smokes is almost 3 times more likely to wheeze than a child in a non smoking home. There's also the possibility that when parents smoke, so will children, setting themselves up for illness in later life.

All studies contributing to the above catalogue of doom are based on cigarette smoking. If however you enjoy a pipe or have a passion for cigars, you can probably take it for granted that the effects of these are a whole lot worse.

## Useful websites/references

**www.chem-tox.com**
A website researching the effect of chemicals and pesticides on health.

**http://www.marchofdimes.com**
**www.babycentre.co.uk**

**http://www.cdc.gov**
Centers for Disease Control and Prevention

## References

**1** Cigarette Smoking During Pregnancy Links to Learning Disabilities Attention Deficit Disorder - A.D.D. Hyperactivity and Behavior Disorders.
By Richard W. Pressinger, M.Ed.
Graduate Research Project - June 1998 - Special Education Department University of South Florida, Tampa, Florida

**2** Auditory Processing Reduced in School Age Children Exposed to Cigarette Smoke. Neurotoxicology and Teratology, Vol. 16(3), 1994
Drs. Joel S. McCartney, Peter A. Fried Department of Psychology, Carleton University, Ontario. Canada (Central Auditory Processing in School-Age Children Prenatally Exposed to Cigarette Smoke).

**3** Smoking During Pregnancy Increases Conduct Disorders
Archives General Psychiatry, 54:670-676, July, 1997
Lauren S. Wakschlag PHD; Benjamin B. Lahey PHD; Rolf Loeber PHD; Stephanie M. Green MS; Rachel A. Gordon MA; Bennett L. Leventhal MD

# 4 Alcohol

Most authorities state that drinking alcohol during pregnancy is something to be avoided. While some advice says that low to moderate alcohol intake is fine, there is increasing evidence showing that drinking any alcohol at all during pregnancy can damage the foetus and give rise to lifelong abnormalities. The Royal College of Physicians recommends that you should avoid alcohol completely while pregnant, whereas the Health Education Authority, the Royal College of Obstetricians and Gynaecologists, and the Food Standards Agency (FSA) all advise low consumption, ie from one or two drinks a week to a maximum of one unit of alcohol per day.

If you're a smoker, drink lots of caffeine or have a poor diet, the effects of alcohol are intensified.

Alcohol can also affect the chances of conception for both of you. Heavy alcohol consumption can reduce a man's testosterone levels, which can lower his sperm count.

Alcohol passes quickly through the placenta to the baby, where it is broken down much more slowly than in an adult. This means that the alcohol level in the child's blood can be higher, and remain for longer, than in the mother's blood.

## Foetal Alcohol Syndrome

Foetal Alcohol Syndrome (FAS) is a rare condition, affecting 1-2 babies in every 1,000 live births. It causes mental and physical disabilities, and classic symptoms include: low birth weight which does not rectify as the child grows, small eyes, small upturned nose, and small, flat cheeks. The internal organs do not form properly, especially the heart, and the brain may be small and abnormally formed. Most babies with FAS will have some degree of mental disability, with poor coordination, low attention span and behavioural problems.

These effects are permanent, and often lead to lifelong psychological problems. Even if the baby does not show signs of FAS, up to 10 times as many babies are born with lesser degrees of damage if the mother has consumed alcohol during pregnancy. This may include some of the symptoms described above, and also Alcohol Related Neurodevelopmental Disorders (ARND).

A report in the Journal of Pediatrics, written by Dr J W Hanson of the Dysmorphology Unit, Department of Pediatrics, University of Washington, describes a study involving 163 middle class, predominantly white children selected from two Seattle, Washington hospitals. They were investigated for any abnormalities by a physician, who was unaware of the parent's drinking background. Afterwards, the assessment was matched with the parental drinking habits, and the following results were determined:

- 10% risk of having abnormal or FAS child if drinking ranged from 2-4 drinks daily
- 19% risk of having abnormal or FAS child if drinking ranged above more than 4 drinks

These are the actual risk figures, meaning if the mother drank 2-4 drinks daily she had a 1 in 10 chance of having an abnormal or FAS child, and if she drank more than 4 drinks daily she had nearly a 1 in 5 chance of having an abnormal or FAS child (1).

Attention, distraction and impulsive behaviour problems were found to occur more often in a study of 475 young school age children whose mothers drank moderate amounts of alcohol during pregnancy. The study, conducted by the University of Washington, used sensitive neurological test measures, called Continuous Performance Tasks (CPT), to determine endurance, persistence, organization, distractibility and impulsivity in these 7 year old children.

One test, for assessing Attention Deficit Disorders, is called the AX-task. The child sits at a computer screen flashing single letters at one second intervals. The child is asked to push a button when the letter "X" appears, but only when it was immediately preceded by the letter "A". The number of errors is then calculated for three different mother alcohol consumption levels (0-3 drinks daily, 3-4 drinks daily, & more than 4 drinks daily) to determine if there was any correlation between the amount of alcohol consumed and the number of errors the child made on the test. The results showed that greater alcohol exposure resulted in far more errors on the AX task.

Tests of distraction were also conducted while the child was taking the CPT tests. There was an 8% distraction rate for the 0-3 drink exposure children, a 14% distraction rate for the 3-4 drink exposure children and a 46% distraction rate for the children whose mothers drank more than 4 drinks per day. Average reaction times were about twice as slow for the more than 3 drink exposure children. In conclusion the researchers stated "This study is important in demonstrating the continuing impact of prenatal alcohol exposure on attention and reaction time in 7 year old children." **(2)**

Part of the brain called the hippocampus is particularly vulnerable during development to the effects of alcohol. However, one study on mice suggests that physical exercise can to some extent alleviate this, and re-stimulate growth. While this doesn't mean you can drink like a fish and then run round the park for an hour a day, it may mean that, if you've consumed alcohol before realising you were pregnant, it's possible that sensible exercise could undo some of the potential damage **(3)**.

There's also evidence to show that, in rats, alcohol consumption during pregnancy can affect the immune system of the offspring for its entire life, even after just one day's drinking in early pregnancy on the part of the mother. While rats are not humans (though some humans are certainly rats), this is worth noting.

Generally, birth defects such as a malformed heart result from drinking in the 1st trimester, while growth problems are associated with drinking in the 3rd. But alcohol consumption at any stage of pregnancy can affect the developing child's brain.

There is an increasing amount of evidence that even one binge drinking session during early pregnancy can adversely affect the child. Research done in 1981 at the University of North Carolina found that although most studies of FAS pinpoint long term heavy use of alcohol, there is a two or three day "critical period" as early as a few weeks after conception when the developing human foetus is especially vulnerable to alcohol effects. Tests on mice that were given just two doses of alcohol equal to about twice the legal limit for humans (they don't say what the legal limit for mice is), 4 hours apart, resulted in foetal malformations in nearly 50% of the offspring **(4)**.

No level of drinking during pregnancy has been proven to be safe. While it is the children of heavily drinking or alcoholic mothers who suffer the most serious abnormalities, even light to moderate drinking can cause nerve damage and physical deformation.

Drinking alcohol during pregnancy also increases the risk of miscarriage, low birthweight and stillbirth, but figures vary as to how much. Some research indicates that heavy drinkers are 2–4 times more likely to have a miscarriage in the 4th to 6th months of pregnancy than non drinking mothers. Other studies claim that the slight increase in miscarriage for women who drink more than three alcoholic drinks per week disappears after the first few weeks, and by the 2nd trimester the risk is the same as for non drinking mothers. Sadly, women have a greater vulnerability to the side effects of booze than men, despite the Sex Equality Act. But if you're hoping to produce the next Einstein, you may wish to give up the tequila slammers and buy a juicer.

## What's a unit?

One unit is equivalent to:
- one half pint of ordinary strength beer, lager or cider
- one quarter pint of strong beer or lager
- one small glass of wine
- one single (pub) measure of spirits
- one small glass of sherry

# References

1 Fetal Alcohol Syndrome Occurs at Moderate Alcohol Levels
Dr. James W. Hanson
Dysmorphology Unit, Department of Pediatrics, University of Washington
Journal of Pediatrics, 92(3):457-460

2 Dr. Ann P. Streissguth, Helen M. Barr, Paul D. Sampson
Department of Psychiatry and Behavioral Sciences
Department of Statistics, Department of Biostatistics, Alcoholism & Drug Institute
Child Development/Mental Retardation, Center of the University of Washington,
Seattle
Neurobehavioral Toxicology and Teratology, 8:717-725, 1986

3 Pubmed: Hippocampus. 2006 Jan 19; [Epub ahead of print]
Hippocampal cell proliferation is reduced following prenatal ethanol exposure
but can be rescued with voluntary exercise.
Redila VA, Olson AK, Swann SE, Mohades G, Webber AJ, Weinberg J, Christie
BR.
Department of Psychology, University of British Columbia, Vancouver

4 Fetal Alcohol Syndrome (FAS) Occurs After One Binge Drinking Episode
Drs. Kathleen K. Sulik, Malcolm C. Johnston and Mary A. Webb
University of North Carolina at Chapel Hill
Science, November 20, 1981

# 5 Recreational drugs

The principal problems with recreational drug use during pregnancy are that the baby's growth can be restricted, and it may also experience withdrawal symptoms after birth, which can hinder emotional bonding. Physical deformities of internal organs, brain and genitalia are possible with certain drugs, and the child may be affected through to adulthood with attention deficit, behavioural and depressive problems.

During the first 10 weeks of pregnancy, most of the organs and body systems of the foetus are formed. Ingestion of drugs (including alcohol) during this phase can cause malformations of the heart, limbs and facial features. Beyond this 10 week period, development of the eyes and nervous system can be impaired, and there is a higher risk of miscarriage or premature birth. The greatest danger is the interference of drugs with the baby's growth: Intra Uterine Growth Retardation (IUGR) results in a low birthweight baby, often born prematurely and/or too small. Such babies need special care and have a much higher risk of severe health problems or death.

If drugs are taken late in pregnancy, the baby may be born addicted and suffer withdrawal symptoms, such as tremors, sleeplessness, muscle spasms, irritability, vomiting and diarrhoea, and joint stiffness. It may have problems suckling. Some experts believe learning difficulties may manifest later in life.

Heavy narcotics use increases the danger of premature birth with such accompanying problems for the infant as low birthweight, breathing difficulties, low blood sugar (hypoglycaemia), and bleeding within the head (intracranial haemorrhage). Mothers who inject narcotics can be infected with the HIV virus if they use dirty or shared needles, and there is a high risk that their babies will also become infected. Both mother and child may then go on to develop AIDS.

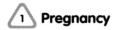 

## Cocaine

This can suppress the mother's appetite, so she doesn't feed either herself or her developing child properly. It causes blood vessels to constrict, increasing heart rate and the blood pressure. This puts greater strain on the mother's body and may slow the baby's growth rate. There's a higher risk of miscarriage, premature labour, stillbirth, and abruptio placentae, where the placenta partially detaches from the uterine wall, causing bleeding which can be life threatening for both mother and child.

Cocaine crosses the placenta and can cause irreversible brain damage or even death. This is more likely to happen if the mother uses cocaine throughout the pregnancy; if she stops in the 1st trimester the risk is reduced. Birth defects associated with cocaine use during pregnancy include abnormalities of the brain, skull, face, eyes, heart, limbs, intestines, genitals and urinary tract. There is also a higher risk of the baby developing cerebral palsy, and visual and hearing impairment. It can have feeding problems and difficulty sleeping. Because the baby can suffer from withdrawal symptoms, it may be jittery, irritable, weepy and unresponsive; some of these problems can last for up to 10 weeks after birth.

Research published in Developmental Psychology Sept 2005 shows that cocaine exposure negatively affects the mother-baby relationship: "Prenatal cocaine and opiate exposure are thought to subtly compromise social and emotional development." Both babies and mothers displayed "negative engagement", ie a lower level of emotional interaction. **(1)**

Another study carried out at the Department of Pediatrics, University of Miami School of Medicine, Florida, was designed to identify associations between cocaine exposure during pregnancy and medical conditions in newborn infants from birth through to hospital discharge. "Cocaine-exposed infants were about 1.2 weeks younger, weighed 536 g less, measured 2.6 cm shorter, and had head circumference 1.5 cm smaller than non-exposed infants." The study also found that problems with the autonomic nervous system were more frequent, and exposed children had more infections. **(2)**

There's no hard and fast data on how high cocaine levels need to be to cause birth defects and other abnormalities. Also, as with alcohol, different people respond differently to the various intoxicants available. Be aware that cocaine is passed on in breast milk in significant amounts, and will continue to affect the baby. Bottle feeding may be the safer option in such circumstances.

## Heroin

Heroin addiction in the mother can cause inter uterine growth retardation (IUGR), leading to premature delivery or stillbirth. Around half of the babies born to heroin addicted women are preterm. As heroin ingestion can be intermittent, a switch to methadone can regulate drug levels and reduce the risks somewhat. Both heroin and methadone can create withdrawal symptoms in the newborn child, including feeding and breathing problems and general distress, and they both cross over into breast milk in small amounts. Again, bottle feeding can be considered as a solution.

Research done at the Women & Children's Hospital, Hull Royal Infirmary, published in September 2005 in the European Journal of Obstetrics, Gynaecology & Reproductive Biology, stated that "The outcome for pregnancy in women who use opiates is complicated by high rates of prematurity and neonatal death." The study observed 110 babies born to 108 mothers. Women who took heroin in later pregnancy were significantly more likely than women who were stabilised on methadone to have a baby who needed morphine (40% versus 19%). These mothers needed a longer hospital stay than women who used only methadone.

## Ecstasy

There isn't much known about the effects of this drug on unborn children, but one study reported by the UK Teratology Information

Service suggested that the incidence of birth defects, mainly of the heart and limbs, was higher than expected. Half the women involved in the research also took other drugs, and drug use was mostly confined to the 1st trimester.

## LSD

The same lack of information goes for LSD (lysergic acid diethylamine) and amphetamines. One piece of research reported that the pure form of LSD didn't cause any foetal abnormalities, and did not increase the risk of miscarriage, though scientifically speaking that's not nearly enough evidence upon which to base an opinion. And the use of street LSD, which is almost never pure, may cause such problems.

## Glue

The organic solvent toluene, commonly found in paint, glue and similar substances, seems to cause similar defects to those produced by alcohol – which itself is an organic solvent.

## PCP

Phencyclidine, or angel dust, has been found to cause withdrawal symptoms in newborns when taken late in pregnancy.

## Cannabis

Again, the most common problem is IUGR (Intra Uterine Growth Retardation) resulting in low birthweight or premature babies. The cannabis issue is clouded (if you'll pardon the pun) by the fact that it is often smoked with tobacco, and it is therefore very difficult to measure which substance is causing the problems.

However, a study carried published in the Journal of Gynaecology Obstetrics & Biological Reproduction (Paris) January 2006, collated scientific research done between 1970-2005. The objective of this review was to examine the association between cannabis use during pregnancy and effects upon growth, cognitive development (memory, attention, executive functions) and behaviour of new-borns, children and teenagers. It found that cannabis use during pregnancy is associated with various neurobehavioural and cognitive outcomes, including "inattention, impulsivity, deficits in learning and memory, and a deficiency in aspects of executive functions." Sadly this last doesn't simply mean that junior may never reach the boardroom, but that he or she has problems physically doing things. **(3)**

Other studies have also found that cannabis use during pregnancy can result in neurological and cognitive problems in the child, including symptoms of ADHD and problems with learning and memory tasks. Also there is evidence to suggest that such cannabis use can lead to depression in the child in later life ("aaw mum, have you been at my skunk again?")

It's also possible that smoking cannabis can affect fertility (scientific studies don't seem to discriminate between smoking weed and taking it in other ways such as eating it). Research done at the University of California, San Diego (I wonder if they had flowers in their hair?) looked at whether cannabis use affected IVF fertilisation. 221 couples were studied, these undergoing either IVF or GIFT (gamete intrafallopian transfer). This showed that women who were heavy users of marijuana had 27% fewer oocytes (egg cells) retrieved, and 1 less embryo transferred than other women. Mothers who had smoked cannabis in the year before fertility treatment had 23% fewer oocytes retrieved. Dads were affected too: those who smoked 11 – 90 times in their lifetime fathered babies that were 15% lighter at birth. Heavy users' offspring were 23% lighter. Mothers who had smoked marijuana more than 10 times had babies who were 17% smaller than those of other women. **(4)**

But just to complicate matters, some women use cannabis during pregnancy to alleviate the symptoms of morning sickness. A Canadian study published in Complementary Therapy Clinical Practice February 2006 examined the subject, carrying out a survey of 79 women who used medical cannabis while pregnant. Of these, 77% had experienced nausea and/or vomiting, 68% had used cannabis to treat the condition, and over 92% rated it as either "extremely effective" or "effective". Maybe this only applies to blissed-out Canadians but it's an interesting piece of research. **(5)**

## References

1 Developmental Psychology 2005 Sept: 41(5):711-22
Cocaine exposure is associated with subtle compromises of infants' and mothers' social-emotional behavior and dyadic features of their interaction in the face-to-face still-face paradigm.
Tronick EZ, Messinger DS, Weinberg MK, Lester BM, Lagasse L, Seifer R, Bauer CR, Shankaran S, Bada H, Wright LL, Poole K, Liu J.
Department of Psychiatry, Harvard Medical School and Child Development Unit, Children's Hospital, Boston,USA.

2 Archive of Pediatric Adolescent Medicine 2005 Sept; 159(9):824-34
Acute neonatal effects of cocaine exposure during pregnancy.
Bauer CR, Langer JC, Shankaran S, Bada HS, Lester B, Wright LL, Krause-Steinrauf H, Smeriglio VL, Finnegan LP, Maza PL, Verter J.
Department of Pediatrics, University of Miami School of Medicine, USA.

3 Journal of Gynaecology Obstetrics Biological Reproduction (Paris) Jan 2006; 35(1):62-70
Short- and long-term consequences of prenatal exposure to cannabis
Karila L, Cazas O, Danel T, Reynaud M.
Departement d'Addictologie et de Psychiatrie, Hopital Paul Brousse, 12, Avenue Paul-Vaillant-Couturier, BP 200, 94804 Villejuif Cedex.

4 Marijuana use affects ART outcome
Source: Human Reproduction 2006; 194: 369-76
Investigating whether marijuana use by men and women affects the outcome of IVF and gamete intrafallopian transfer. Hillary Klonoff-Cohen (University of California, San Diego) and colleagues.

5 Complementary Therapy Clinical Practice 2006 Feb;12(1):27-33 epub 2005 Dec.
Survey of medicinal cannabis use among childbearing women: Patterns of its use in pregnancy and retroactive self-assessment of its efficacy against 'morning sickness'.
Westfall RE, Janssen PA, Lucas P, Capler R.
Michael Smith Foundation for Health Research Postdoctoral Fellow, Department of Sociology, University of Victoria, Canada.

# 6 Medication

No matter how organic, natural, chemical free and hemp woven you may want your pregnancy to be, there are times when you need medication and can't safely do without it. So how will it affect junior?

## Anti-depressants

Selective serotonin reuptake inhibitors (SSRIs) have gained wide acceptance in the treatment of mental disorders in pregnant women.

Paroxetine hydrochloride (Seroxat) is often prescribed for maternal depression, panic disorder and obsessive compulsive disorder (OCD). It crosses the placenta, and although it doesn't appear to increase teratogenic risk (foetal malformation in the 1st trimester), there have been case reports of neonatal withdrawal. Symptoms can last up to one month but are usually temporary.

One study examined "Perinatal Outcome Following Third Trimester Exposure to Paroxetine". The researchers wanted to know if the drug affected the behaviour of the newborn baby. It was a prospective, controlled cohort study (2 groups of subjects, one exposed to the drug being tested, the other not). Of the 55 newborns exposed to paroxetine in late gestation, 12 had complications requiring intensive treatment and a prolonged stay in hospital. The most common disorder was respiratory distress, followed by hypoglycaemia and jaundice. In the comparison group, only 3 babies experienced complications. Only 3rd trimester exposure to the drug was associated with neonatal distress. [1]

A study done earlier, in 1996: Birth Outcomes in Pregnant Women Taking Fluoxetine (Prozac) gave similar results, examining 228 pregnant women taking fluoxetine in comparison with a control group of 254 non-medicated women. The results showed that the babies of women on fluoxetine in the 3rd trimester had lower birth weight, were shorter, and had an increased risk of perinatal complications. **(2)**

This research is backed up by a study on "Neonate Characteristics After Maternal Use of Antidepressants in Late Pregnancy" published in April 2004. This found that for 997 babies born to mothers who had used prescribed anti depressants, there was an increased risk of preterm birth, low birth weight, respiratory distress, neonatal convulsions and hypoglycaemia (this last especially regarding use of tricyclics). **(3)**

In November 2005, tests done on 10 women taking nortriptyline and seven taking clomipramine found that "Obstetrical complications, such as pre-term delivery and pregnancy induced hypertension, were increased compared to the national average". **(4)**

However, a paper published in CMAJ in 2005 by 5 experts, expressed concern that untreated depression in pregnant women was more dangerous than any slight and temporary risk to the baby. The authors felt that the American FDA (Food & Drug Administration) had been precipitate in issuing instructions to manufacturers of anti-depressants to give warnings about perinatal complications associated with their products. Doctors were also advised to taper the dosage of anti-depressants in pregnant women during the last trimester so the foetus would not receive any drug for at least 8-10 days before birth. The authors of the paper state: "We believe those recommendations are only partially evidence-based and may put the depressed mother-to-be and her baby at an unreasonable health risk." And: "When used at recommended dosages during pregnancy, neither SSRIs nor SNRIs (serotonin-nor-epinephrine reuptake inhibitors) have shown any evidence of teratogenic effects."

## Benzodiazepines

These include: diazepam (Valium) alprazolam (Xanax) and lorazepam (Ativan).

Benzodiazepines, usually prescribed for anxiety related problems, do cross the placenta, and there is a risk that if you take them during the first 3 months of pregnancy they can cause malformations. They also carry into breast milk. Symptoms seen in newborns include: limpness, getting very cold, breathing problems, and sleeping too much to feed properly. The baby can also suffer withdrawal symptoms.

## Asthma medication

If you have asthma, then you may find that it changes during your pregnancy. Roughly 1/3rd of women find it improves, a 1/3rd that it gets worse, while for 1/3rd it stays the same. It is important to maintain your medication while pregnant, as a reduction in your breathing capacity can lead to the baby not getting enough oxygen. So you'll want to know if your drugs are safe for your baby. Surprisingly little research has been done on this, but there are concerns that beta-2 agonists like albuterol (aka Ventolin, salbutamol,and Epipen auto injector) can cause cleft palate and other skull and facial deformities.

Several animal studies have shown that albuterol does cause these defects, but the doses used were far higher than any human would (or probably could) inhale – up to 600 times more in some cases (and if you took that amount of almost anything it would be bound to have some sort of undesirable effect).

However, in a study cited on the Internet drug index rxlist.com, a mouse trial showed that where the dose of albuterol, given subcutaneously, was the same as the maximum recommended human daily inhaled dose, 4.5% of the mouse foetuses showed cleft palate formation (5 out of 111). At 8.0 times more, 9.3% (10 out of 108) had the defect.

There are several studies that back up the results of the one above, some done on rabbits but none on humans. Other asthma treatments such as isoproterenol and metaproterenol have similar results to albuterol, while terbutaline has been shown to be safe in both animal and human tests. Epinephrine (adrenalin) however, which is used for emergency allergic reactions, has been shown to cause birth defects in humans – but again, you don't take it every day in huge doses, and staying alive is a prerequisite to giving birth if you're a mammal.

Intravenous salbutamol (ventolin) is sometimes used in the management of premature labour, as it acts as a uterine muscle relaxant. Inhaled salbutamol should not affect your pregnancy in this manner, but check with your doctor if you're concerned. The propellant used in your Ventolin inhaler is non CFC HFA 134a, and this has been found to be non toxic in animal studies where the subjects were exposed to the propellant daily for over 2 years.

## Corticosteroids

These are drugs that mimic certain hormones that your body naturally produces. They are prescribed to control allergic reactions topically (on the skin) or via inhaler for conditions such as asthma. There's not a huge amount of research on these regarding pregnancy, but a study and a meta analysis (a gathering together of the results of a number of studies to get the bigger picture) reported on Bandolier (a medical research website) looked at birth defects after maternal exposure to corticosteroids.

First the study: a group of 184 women had been using prednisone for 21 weeks, at an average daily dose of 27mg. 75% were exposed to the drug during the 1st trimester. These corticosteroid users were more likely than the control group to be smokers. The non-user control group consisted of 188 women.

The number of live births was similar in each group, as was the number of miscarriages, foetal deaths and stillbirths. The babies born to the medicated mothers were smaller (mean: 3,112g versus 3,428g), were born earlier (mean: 38 weeks versus 39.5 weeks) and were more likely to be premature (27 babies versus 9). "Despite these differences, the majority of babies in both groups were an appropriate weight for their gestational age. There was no difference in the number of major abnormalities between the groups (4 out of 111 exposed babies; 3 out of 172 unexposed babies)."

The meta analysis consisted of 10 studies (6 cohort and 4 case control). Case control means identifying patients who have experienced birth defects, and control patients who haven't, and looking at their case histories to see if they have been exposed to the drug in question.

A total of 51,470 women in the cohort studies, and 71,705 in the case control studies were involved. After adjustments for accuracy, the cohort study showed a significant risk of major defects. Cleft palate was the most common, with 3 out of 390 babies affected. There were no cases among the 708 non exposed babies. The four case control studies showed that there was an increased risk of oral clefts when the foetus was exposed to corticosteroids during the 1st trimester.

The overall message of this piece of research states: "The risk of oral clefts increases threefold in foetuses exposed to corticosteroids during the first trimester." **(6)**

Scientifically there's a question that you must always ask in these circumstances: "Does the potential benefit justify the potential risk?" In other words, you have to decide if the need for the medication is such that, if you did not take it, you would be putting yourself and your child at significant risk.

## NSAIDs

Non Steroidal Anti Inflammatory Drugs (NSAIDs) are thought to be one of the most commonly prescribed drugs during pregnancy. They include: diclofenac (Voltarol), ibuprofen (Nurofen, Advil), ketoprofen (Oruvail, Orudis), nabumetone (Relifex), naproxen (Synflex, Naprosyn), piroxicam (Feldene).

Some newer NSAIDs are called cox-2 inhibitors, such as celecoxib (Celebrex), Etoricoxib (Arcoxia).

According to the Bulletin on the Rheumatic Diseases Volume 51, Number 9: Anti-Rheumatic Drugs in Pregnancy: "All NSAIDs are contraindicated in the third trimester because they can promote premature closure of the ductus arteriosus, which will result in pulmonary hypertension for the foetus. However, some studies have shown reversal of the ductal constriction within 48 hours of stopping the NSAID." **(7)** Other contraindications associated with the use of NSAIDs throughout pregnancy include reduction in the amount of amniotic fluid, increased risk of foetal haemorrhage, and post partum (birth) bleeding. Some can bring on premature labour.

However, a study by Ostensen & Ostensen: Safety of Nonsteroidal Anti-inflammatory Drugs in Pregnant Patients with Rheumatic Diseases compared 2 groups of pregnant women – 88 in total – one of which took NSAIDs throughout pregnancy. This study showed no difference between the 2 groups with regard to pregnancy outcome, duration of labour or neonatal health. **(8)**

A paper entitled "Exposure to Non-steroidal Anti-inflammatory Drugs During Pregnancy and Risk of Miscarriage: Population Based Cohort Study" published in 2003 interviewed 1055 pregnant women about their use of NSAIDs, aspirin and paracetamol during their pregnancy. Prenatal NSAID use was associated with an 80% increased risk of miscarriage, and aspirin use was similarly associated with such an increased risk. Paracetamol however had no such association. The study did stress that further research was required to confirm these findings. **(9)**

## Aspirin

Aspirin (acetylsalicylic acid, salicylic acid) in low doses (50mg) can help women at high risk from pre eclampsia. It is an anti-platelet drug, meaning it reduces the "stickiness" of blood. For this reason it's often taken by people with a higher risk of heart disease as it thins the blood and helps it flow more easily. Of course the downside of this is that you'll bleed like a stuck pig if you cut yourself.

For healthy women aspirin would seem to be safe to take during pregnancy as an occasional analgesic. A few scientific studies suggest that taking aspirin around the time of conception and in early pregnancy is associated with an increased risk of miscarriage (see NSAIDs above). There may also be a higher risk of placental abruption (where part of the placenta comes away from the uterine wall).

A meta analysis on aspirin consumption during the 1st trimester of pregnancy and congenital abnormalities reported in the American Journal of Obstetrics and Gynecology 2002 looked at 22 studies, 1 randomised and the rest either case control or cohort studies. The conclusion was that there was no association between aspirin use and overall abnormalities, though there was a small increased risk for gastroschisis (imperfect closure of the baby's abdomen, usually leaving a hole near the belly button where bowel protrudes) in a small number of pregnancies. (The occurrence of gastroschisis has been steadily increasing over the past 10 years and is now seen in around 4.4 per 10,000 births.) The studies did not have confirmed diagnosis, and maternal disease may have contributed to the result observed). **(10)**

## Paracetamol

Aka acetaminophen, APAP, Panodol, Tylenol. The biggest study done on paracetamol use in pregnancy in the UK is part of the ALSPAC study (Avon Longitudinal Study of Pregnancy and Childhood) involving over 12,000 women. Presented in 1996, this research concluded that neither pregnancy nor infant development was adversely affected by normal use of the drug. 43.6% of the mothers in the study took paracetamol during the first 6 months of their pregnancy.

Dr Shaheen, lead author of the ALSPAC study, has gone on to examine this finding with relation to asthma in later childhood: in "Prenatal Paracetamol Exposure and Risk of Asthma and Elevated Immunoglobulin E in Childhood" (2005) the study team measured associations of paracetamol and aspirin use in late pregnancy (20-

32 weeks) with asthma, hayfever, eczema and wheezing in the off-spring at 69-81 months.

They found that use of paracetamol, but not aspirin, in late pregnancy was positively associated with asthma, comparing children whose mothers took paracetamol 'sometimes' and 'most days/daily' with those whose mothers never took it. The proportion of asthma attributable to paracetamol use in late pregnancy, assuming a causal relation, was 7%. They concluded that "Paracetamol exposure in late gestation may cause asthma, wheezing and elevated IgE (immunoglobulin E, an antibody triggered by allergies) in children of school age." **(11)**

An article on Perinatology.com: Drugs in Pregnancy & Breastfeeding, synthesises results from several research studies. 3 studies totalling more than 10,000 newborns who were exposed to paracetamol during the 1st trimester found no link between the drug and major malformations.

There may however be a problem when paracetamol is used alongside pseudoephedrine, as in cough, cold and analgesic medications. Some research showed an increased risk of gastroschisis. A retrospective study examined the mothers of 206 babies with gastroschisis and 126 mothers of babies with both gastroschisis and small intestinal atresia (SIA). These had an increased risk of having been exposed to paracetamol during pregnancy. The risk for gastroschisis was higher again when the mother had taken a combination of paracetamol and pseudoephedrine.

## Useful websites/references

**http://www.jr2.ox.ac.uk/bandolier**
Excellent medical research site

**http://www.besttreatments.co.uk**
Advice for patients from the British Medical Journal (BMJ)

**www.perinatology.com**
US scientific site on foetal care

# Other references

1 Archives of Pediatrics & Adolescent Medicine vol 156:1129-1132 no 11 2002
Perinatal Outcome Following Third Trimester Exposure to Paroxetine
Adriana Moldovan Costei, MD; Eran Kozer, MD; Tommy Ho, MD, FRCPC; Shinya
Ito, MD; Gideon Koren, MD, FRCPC
From the Motherisk program, Division of Clinical Pharmacology/Toxicology, the
Hospital for Sick Children, and the University of Toronto, Canada.

2 New England Journal of Medicine vol 335:1010-1015 Oct 1996 no 14
Birth Outcomes in Pregnant Women Taking Fluoxetine
Christina D. Chambers, B.A., Kathleen A. Johnson, B.A., Lyn M. Dick, B.A.,
Robert J. Felix, B.A., and Kenneth Lyons Jones, M.D.
From the Department of Pediatrics, Division of Dysmorphology and Teratology,
University of California–San Diego, La Jolla.

3 Neonate Characteristics After Maternal Use of Antidepressants in Late
Pregnancy
Bengt Källén, MD, PhD
Archive of Pediatric and Adolescent Medicine. 2004;158:312-316. vol 158 no 4
April 2004

4 Biological Psychiatry 2005 Nov 1; epub Copyright © 2005 Society of Biological
Psychiatry Published by Elsevier Inc.
Placental Passage of Tricyclic Antidepressants.
Loughhead AM, Stowe ZN, Newport DJ, Ritchie JC, Devane CL, Owens MJ.
Department of Psychiatry and Behavioral Sciences (AML, ZNS, DJN, JCR, MJO).

5 CMAJ • May 24, 2005; 172 (11). doi:10.1503/cmaj.1041100.
© 2005 CMA Media Inc. or its licensors (Canadian Medical Association Journal)
Commentary: Is maternal use of selective serotonin reuptake inhibitors in the
third trimester of pregnancy harmful to neonates?
Gideon Koren, Doreen Matsui, Adrienne Einarson, David Knoppert and Meir
Steiner
From the Motherisk Program, The Hospital for Sick Children and University of
Toronto, Toronto, Ont. (Koren, Einarson); the Ivey Chair in Molecular Toxicology
(Koren), the Department of Pediatrics, University of Western Ontario, London,
Ont. (Koren, Matsui, Knoppert); and the Departments of Psychiatry and
Behavioural Neurosciences and of Obstetrics and Gynecology, McMaster
University, Hamilton, Ont. (Steiner)

6 L Park-Wyllie et al. Birth defects after maternal exposure to corticosteroids:
prospective cohort study and meta-analysis of epidemiological studies.
Teratology 2000 62: 385-392.

**7** Moise KJ, Huhta JC, Sharif DS, et al. Indomethacin in the treatment of preterm labor: effects on the fetal ductus arterosus. New England Journal of Medicine 1988;319:327-31.

**8** Ostensen M, Ostensen H: Safety of nonsteroidal anti-inflammatory drugs in pregnant patients with rheumatic diseases. Journal of Rheumatology 1996;23:1045-9.

**9** British Medical Journal 2003;327:368 (16 August), doi:10.1136/bmj.327.7411.368
Exposure to non-steroidal anti-inflammatory drugs during pregnancy and risk of miscarriage: population based cohort study
De-Kun Li, epidemiologist, Liyan Liu, programmer analyst, Roxana Odouli, research associate.
Division of Research, Kaiser Foundation Research Institute, Oakland, California, USA

**10** E Kozer et al. Aspirin consumption during the first trimester of pregnancy and congenital abnormalities: a meta-analysis. American Journal of Obstetrics and Gynecology 2002 187: 1623-1630.

**11** Comment in: Clinical and Experimental Allergy 2005 Jun;35(6):700-2
Prenatal paracetamol exposure and risk of asthma and elevated immunoglobulin E in childhood.
Shaheen SO, Newson RB, Henderson AJ, Headley JE, Stratton FD, Jones RW, Strachan DP; ALSPAC Study Team.
Department of Public Health Sciences, Guy's, King's and St Thomas' School of Medicine, King's College London, London, UK.

# 7 Exercise

It used to be thought that pregnant women should lie down with their feet up for 9 months. Alas, times change, and although you're not expected to run a marathon 3 days before your due date, neither are you expected to remain inert.

For centuries women have had to do a full day's hard physical work while pregnant: all those apocryphal stories about sturdy peasants popping a baby out under a bush and then returning to ox wrestling or sheep juggling are not so far from the truth.

In parts of Indonesia, when a wife becomes pregnant it's her husband who takes it easy, and the moment she's given birth she has to get up and minister to him, he having undergone sympathetic labour pains and being in dire need of a cup of tea. I refrain from comment in the interests of the health of my spleen.

So should you exercise and, if so, how much? And are there any reasons not to?

## Physical changes

Your body does weird things when you're pregnant. Your joints loosen, you may get toothache, hair can become thinner while everything else gets fatter, your heart rate increases and you make more blood, vein capacity increases too, you sweat more, your metabolic rate rises, you need to wee all the time, you might retain fluid (oedema) while needing to drink more water, and you eventually turn green and become radioactive (spot the fib). You may discover the delights of haemorrhoids, bleeding gums, heartburn, varicose veins, itching, headaches and swollen fingers and toes. Exercising can help alleviate most of these and will improve your mood too.

## Benefits

Exercise releases endorphins and serotonin in your brain, making you feel good and reducing your chances of becoming a growly bear. It can relieve constipation by accelerating movement in your intestine. It may help you to sleep better, both because of physical exertion and by relieving stress. During pregnancy your joints become looser due to a hormone called relaxin, and exercise activates the synovial fluid that keeps them lubricated. You'll look better too, because blood flow to your skin is increased, giving you that sought after glow. If you exercised before getting pregnant, you'll gain less fat during the pregnancy (average weight gain from pre- to post-pregnancy is 10 – 12lbs).

As with most other physical challenges, strong muscles and a fit heart will help your labour and delivery, and if things go slowly you'll have increased endurance to help you cope. Exercise will also help your posture and muscle tone, and can prevent backache. You will be able to carry the extra weight of a baby and all that liquid more easily, and will be less likely to experience swollen ankles. It will be easier to lose any weight gain afterwards too. And after 9 months of occupation, your body will become your own again, and exercise is a good way to take back possession.

A study called: "Effects of a back-pain-reducing program during pregnancy for Korean women: A non-equivalent control-group pretest-posttest study" (not known for their snappy titles, these scientists) took 2 groups of women, 27 who didn't have any back therapy, and 29 who did. Data were collected from both groups at 3 points: beforehand, then 6 and 12 weeks into the programme. Intensity of back pain, functional limitation and anxiety were measured. Conclusion: "At 12 weeks after intervention [exercise], the intensity of back pain experienced by the intervention group was significantly lower than that of the control group." And "Promoting good posture and regular exercise can be recommended as a method to relieve back pain in pregnant women." **(1)**

Another study done in Zurich in 2005 wanted to find out if water based exercise such as aqua fitness classes was useful for pregnancy leg oedema (swollen ankles). The 9 women tested were in normal healthy 2nd or 3rd trimester pregnancy. Leg circumference was measured beforehand (or should that be foot?). After a single session of pool based exercise, mean left leg volume had decreased by 112 ml from 1665 to 1553 ml, and right leg volume by 84 ml from 1665 to 1581 ml. The researchers concluded that "A single immersion exercise session is a safe, effective, and enjoyable complement, or alternative, to compression stockings for reduction of gestational dependent oedema." **(2)**

Research indicates that exercise during pregnancy is good for your baby too. A South Korean animal study examined the effect of daily exercise – in this case swimming – on the short term memory and nerve generation of baby rats. The researchers found that when the mother rats did 10 minutes swimming every day until birth, their offspring showed enhanced short term memory abilities. "The present results have clearly shown that maternal swimming by rats during pregnancy enhances the memory of the rats' offspring by increasing neurogenesis [nerve growth]." So if you want a baby that's as smart as a rat, you know what to do **(3)**.

There has been concern that exercise increases norepinephrine (adrenalin) and prostaglandin output, and that this could in theory stimulate uterine activity and premature birth. Some occupational (ie work) activity may carry a small risk of this happening. But other studies suggest that prolonged standing, ie at certain types of work, is the critical factor: this can decrease heart rate by as much as 18%. Research focusing on recreational exercise tends to confirm a beneficial effect for both mother and baby.

What position you're in can have an effect on your heart rate too. After the first 3 months, lying flat on your back can decrease cardiac output by an average of 9%. The expanding uterus can compress veins and restrict blood flow to the heart. You can remedy this by lying on your side.

# ⚠ Pregnancy

Unpleasantnesses such as nausea and fatigue can be alleviated by exercise, and self esteem is improved. Generally, the same benefits you'd get from exercising when not pregnant apply when you're gravid, with added extras such as symptom relief and a baby that's good at mazes and finding cheese.

Pioneers such as James Clapp., M.D. and Elizabeth Noble have shown through their research that when the mother exercises regularly it enables an easier pregnancy and delivery. In fact, Dr. Clapp found through a study of 500 pregnant women that those who exercised delivered a healthier baby with a stronger foetal heart rate. Even more attractive is the finding that of the women who exercised, time spent in labour was shortened by about a third, with 65% of the women delivering in 4 hours or less.

## References

1   International Journal of Nursing Studies 2005 Dec 28; Epub ahead of print.

Effects of a back-pain-reducing program during pregnancy for Korean women:
A non-equivalent control-group pretest-posttest study.
Shim MJ, Lee YS, Oh HE, Kim JS.
Gwangju Health College, South Korea.

2   Response of pregnancy leg oedema to a single immersion exercise session.
Sabine Hartmann Renate Huch
Perinatal Physiology Research Unit, Department of Obstetrics, Zurich University
Hospital, Zurich, Switzerland.

3   Brain & Development 2005 Dec 17; Epub ahead of print. Elsevier Science Direct.
Maternal swimming during pregnancy enhances short-term memory and neurogenesis in the hippocampus of rat pups.
a:Hee-Hyuk Lee, a:Hong Kim, a:Jin-Woo Lee, a:Young-Sick Kim, a:Hye-Young
Yang, a:Hyun-Kyung Chang, a:Taeck-Hyun Lee, a:Min-Chul Shin, a:Myoung-
Hwa Lee, a:Mal-Soon Shin, a:b:Sooyeon Park, a:c:Seungsoo Baek and
a:Chang-Ju Kim
a:Department of Physiology, College of Medicine, Kyung Hee University, #1
Hoigi-dong, Dongdaemoon-gu, Seoul 130-701, South Korea
b:College of Physical Education, Kyung Hee University, Yongin-si, Gyeonggi-do,
South Korea
c:Department of Physical Education, College of Education, Seoul National
University, Seoul, South Korea

# General information

American Family Physician. Published by American Academy of Family Physicians.
Vol 57 no 8, April 15 1998.

Exercise During Pregnancy

Thomas W Wang, M.D., director of the Primary Care Sports Medicine Fellowship at
the Department of Family Practice at MacNeal Hospital, Berwyn, Illinois.

Barbara S Apgar, M.D., clinical associate professor in the Department of Family
Practice at the University of Michigan Medical School, Ann Arbor, Michigan.


Article from WebMD feature archive.
Pregnancy no excuse for inactivity. By Gay Frankenfield RN

The Physician & Sports Medicine vol 27 no 8 August 1999

Exercise During Pregnancy Safe and Beneficial for Most
Raul Artal, MD, with Carl Sherman
Series Editor: Nicholas A. DiNubile, MD

# 8 Toxoplasmosis

Many pregnant women are concerned about the dangers of catching toxoplasmosis, but in fact by the age of 30, 3 out of every 10 people have had it and most likely never realised it. And once you've had it you're immune for life. 1 in every 50,000 babies born per year has toxoplasmosis, which is a very low figure. The earlier in pregnancy infection occurs, the worse effect it can have on the unborn foetus. The scare stories about this disease are centred upon its effect on the developing child, and this includes hydrocephalus (fluid in the brain), brain damage leading to epilepsy and mental retardation, and eye damage which can cause partial or total sight loss.

In anyone except an unborn child the symptoms are flu-like and relatively mild. It is caused by a parasite called toxoplasma which is found in raw meat, goat's milk products and cat faeces and is killed by cooking or pasteurisation (although I don't recommend this for the faeces). Uncooked foodstuffs like Parma ham may contain toxoplasma, and it can also be present in soil, so may contaminate unwashed root and salad vegetables.

The likelihood of you catching toxoplasmosis from your cat is not high; it's more usually caught from something you've eaten. Sensible precautions are the order of the day:

- Wash all fresh veg thoroughly
- Wash hands, chopping boards & utensils after cutting meat or poultry
- Get someone else to empty the cat litter tray
- Wear gloves when gardening
- Don't let raw meat drip onto other food in the fridge
- Cook all meat thoroughly until juices run clear

If you're worried that you might have caught toxoplasmosis you can ask your doctor to do a blood test to see if you have antibodies. If you do, you've either already had it and thus are safely immune, or you may recently have caught it. Which is confusing (no antibodies means no immunity so you need to take especial care). If you catch toxoplasmosis while pregnant there's a 40% chance of passing it on to your unborn child. To find out if the baby has toxoplasmosis, a sample of umbilical cord blood or amniotic fluid can be taken. Treatment with antibiotics asap can greatly reduce the possibility that your baby will become infected.

## Useful websites/references

**http://www.shef.ac.uk**
University of Sheffield, the Centre for Pregnancy Nutrition

**http://www.jr2.ox.ac.uk/bandolier**
Excellent, readable scientific website

**http://www.marchofdimes.com**
**http://www.babycentre.co.uk**
**http://www.cdc.gov**
Centers for Disease Control and Prevention

# 9 Flying

Flying while pregnant is usually safe and problem free – unless you're a Quidditch player – and as ever, common sense is your most valuable commodity. If you are in a high-risk group, for example having a multiple pregnancy, are diabetic or significantly overweight, have an increased chance of thrombosis, premature labour or bleeding, or you're prone to livening things up by screaming "oh god we're all going to die!!!" then it may be wiser to postpone air travel until you are safely delivered.

Being in the 1st or 3rd trimester increases the risk of miscarriage or premature labour respectively, whether you're on the ground or above it. As it's extremely inconvenient giving birth in a cramped aircraft seat with your legs sprawled awkwardly across the aisle, you need to think about the necessity of your flight (if only for the sake of your modesty).

## Cabin pressure

This is lower than normal air pressure and can fluctuate during the flight, placing added strain on your heart and lungs as they have to work harder to provide you with oxygen (or what passes for it in some planes where they just recycle the cabin air, ensuring that everyone has an opportunity to catch passenger no. 52's Nepalese Yak flu). If you have high blood pressure, a history of blood clots, or circulatory problems, you are in the high-risk category. Bear in mind also that in the 3rd trimester your blood pressure can increase anyway.

## Radiation

The higher you fly, the more radiation there is, so long haul flights increase your exposure. Or rather that of your foetus, which is much more sensitive to it than you are. On average, a person is normally exposed to 2.6 millisieverts (mSv) of ionising radiation per year. A frequent flyer can receive up to 4.6 mSv, compared to a nuclear worker's 3.6 mSv. The European annual limit for air crew is 6.00 mSv, which translates as 200 hours flying time. So unless you are going to fly long haul twice a week for the entire duration of your pregnancy the risk is considered minimal.

## Dehydration

Aircraft cabins are much drier than the normal atmosphere you breathe, so drink lots of water (no alcohol) during your flight. Despite the fact that this will mean frequent visits to the pixie loo (that tiny cupboard you'll have to reverse into or risk getting your bump jammed against the sink) it will keep you hydrated, keep your airways moist thus reducing your chances of catching the Yak flu, and make you get up and down a lot, hopefully avoiding the next little problem...

## DVT

Deep vein thrombosis occurs when, usually through inactivity, a clot forms in a leg vein, breaks up, and travels to somewhere much more serious like the lungs, causing a pulmonary embolism – which is among the top 10 things to avoid on holiday. DVT is considered the biggest air travel risk for pregnant women, who are 5 times more likely to develop it. The recommended precautions are: wear flight socks, keep your feet and ankles flexing and get up to walk about every half hour or so. Business Class is roomier than Economy, but the risk of DVT is the same in either, despite what the tabloids may tell you.

Symptoms to watch out for include pain, tenderness and swelling, with possible discolouration: the leg can turn either pale blue or a reddish purple colour. If the thrombosis develops in a thigh vein, as is common in pregnancy, the whole leg may become swollen. Oddly, left legs are more prone to DVT than right legs due to more complicated wiring.

Treatment involves an anticoagulant: Low Molecular Weight

heparin (LMW heparin) which has a very low-risk of side effects. It's injected under the skin, or via a small pump that regulates the dose, and doesn't cross the placenta or pass into breast milk. The other treatment for DVT is warfarin, which is rat poison and not suitable for pregnant women (or rats) as it does cross the placenta and can lead to developmental problems in the foetus.

## Food

Some might argue that eating airline food is never a good idea, but for you it may present particular problems. Reheated food carries a higher risk of contamination, and although airlines take great care not to kill off their passengers with botulism or salmonella, you might want to take a packed lunch if you're concerned about this. On a budget carrier this may be a necessity anyway, unless you're happy to blow half your holiday spending money on a BLT (boring, limp, tasteless) sandwich and undrinkable tea from the trolley.

## Vaccinations

Some exotic destinations offer a wide choice of equally exotic diseases for you to catch, so check to see if you'll need vaccinations before you go. These are not a good idea as they can cause complications for both you and your baby, so if you really do have to go to a malaria infested swamp for your holiday you can get an exemption from your doctor. It's also worth noting that some countries may not let you in if you are heavily pregnant.

## Time limits

Tell the airline you're pregnant; they will put you in a roomier seat and the crew will be extra lovely to you which is terrific. Airlines all have their own rules about carrying pregnant passengers so check this out before booking. In general you can fly until the 24th/28th week, but beyond that you require a letter or medical certificate from your GP or midwife confirming your expected delivery date, their approval for you to fly, and the excellent state of your health. Past the 32nd/36th week airlines will generally not carry you at all. Long haul flights (8 hours or more) restrict you to 28 weeks. Some airlines will allow you to travel very late in your pregnancy for compassionate reasons – keeping that hair appointment is not serious enough I'm afraid – but they will insist you are accompanied by a doctor or nurse. It is therefore very important to check the policy for the carrier you will travel with, for both your outward and return dates.

## Baby

Once your baby is no longer travelling as tum luggage – and you didn't give birth in the actual aircraft – different rules apply. Your bundle of joy must be at least 2 days old and preferably 7 or more before being allowed on a plane. You may need a letter from your GP stating that it's OK for you both to fly. If you are within 48 hours of giving birth, or 10 days of having a Caesarean, the airline will probably not carry you.

## Useful websites/references

http://www.thrombosis-charity.org.uk
http://airtravel.about.com
Summarises the policies of several major airlines regarding pregnancy.

http://www.britishairways.com
British Airways

www.bupa.co.uk
Go to Health Information and use searchterm "flying while pregnant"

## Other references

South African Medical Journal 2003; 93(7): 522-8
The BEST study –a prospective study to compare business class versus economy class air travel as a cause of thrombosis.
Jacobson BF, Munster M, Smith A, Burnand KG, Carter A, Abdool-Carrim AT, Marcos E, Becker PJ, Rogers T, le Roux D, Calvert-Evers JL, Nel MJ, Brackin R, Veller M. Newcombe, R.

# 10  Ultrasound

This is the first screening test you will be offered, but you don't have to have any scans or tests if you don't want to. The first scan is to confirm the date your pregnancy began and is usually performed at 10-13 weeks. It's done by a trained sonographer and involves you having a full bladder and lots of chilly gel being put on your stomach. High frequency sound waves (2-13 mHz) are directed through the uterus which pass through liquid but bounce back off the foetus.

If you are significantly overweight or the baby is too deep in your pelvis, an ultrasound will not produce clear images, so a vaginal scan may be necessary. This involves a long thin transducer placed inside the vagina, and will give a much clearer picture of the foetus.

## Anomaly scan

This is a screening test, done at 20 weeks to check that the foetus is developing properly. You should be given information about what the scan is for, so you can decide whether or not you want one. Your baby will be about 8 inches long now, and will look like a proper little human being. Its sex can be determined at this stage, though not all hospitals will give you this information. The sonographer will check the baby's internal organs and skeletal structure, and measure skull circumference and diameter, femur length and abdominal circumference. As this is a detailed scan it takes around 20 minutes.

The kinds of problems this scan can pick up include spina bifida (exposed spinal cord); anencephaly (top of the skull missing); major limb defects ie missing or very short; defects of the abdominal wall; major kidney problems. It may also pick up diaphragmatic hernia, hydrocephalus (excess fluid in the brain), and possible signs of a risk of Down's syndrome. There are some abnormalities that won't be visible yet, such as heart defects and bowel obstructions.

The scan can also reveal other things: a blighted ovum means that conception occurred as usual and the egg implanted in the uterus, but no embryo has developed. A missed miscarriage shows an embryo with no heartbeat, meaning that it started to develop but then stopped, and hasn't been expelled by the body in the usual way. You may discover the presence of one or more placental lakes. These are pools or collections of blood either on the surface or inside the placenta. Almost all placentas develop these by the 3rd trimester and there is no evidence that they are a problem.

Single umbilical artery (SUA) may show up on a scan at this time, and means that instead of the usual 1 vein and 2 arteries inside the umbilical cord, there's only a vein and 1 artery. This can be associated with congenital abnormalities such as heart, skeletal, intestinal and kidney problems, so the sonographer will take a very careful look at these. SUA is also a marker for chromosomal abnormalities but, as with other markers, if it's on its own there is unlikely to be a problem.

Amniotic band syndrome involves threads or bands in the amniotic fluid. In early pregnancy there are 2 separate layers of membrane. The outer one is the chorion, and the inner is the amnion. By week 16 these should have fused, but it is possible for the amnion to tear or rupture before this happens. If this occurs, the amnion can form threads that wrap around the baby. This can disrupt the blood supply, potentially leading to significant abnormalities, but it is very rare.

Bleeding in the 1st trimester is quite common, and as long as it's just spotting it isn't usually indicative of anything scary. If the bleeding is a little heavier, it may be due to blood clots under the placenta (retroplacental or chorionic haematoma). If the affected area is small, the blood is usually reabsorbed and no harm done. If however the area is large, this may increase the chance of miscarriage, and a scan will be suggested to see how things are going. If there is bleeding at any time during the pregnancy that is more than spotting, it should be checked out straight away.

If you do miscarry it doesn't necessarily mean you'll have any problems with future pregnancies – most healthy women go on to achieve a full term pregnancy next time.

## Ultrasound markers

These are controversial. Sometimes babies with chromosomal abnormalities show signs called ultrasound markers. The problem is that lots of normal babies also show these markers. A marker is a slight difference in anatomy, and in a normal baby these resolve themselves without any interference. But because these markers may sometimes be a sign of an abnormality, they are taken note of. If there are two or more, you may be offered further testing so that a diagnosis can be made. This will mean collecting some of the baby's cells via CVS (chorionic villus sampling) or amniocentesis. The four most common markers are choroid plexus cysts (CPCs), renal pelvic dilatation (RPD), echogenic bowel, and echogenic foci in the ventricles of the heart (golf balls).

Similarly, physical differences such as short limbs, short or bent little fingers, and a gap between the big and other toes have been suggested as markers for Down's syndrome, but as lots of normal babies have these too, such markers cannot be relied upon.

About 15% of ultrasound scans need to be repeated, usually for perfectly innocuous reasons. If there is a problem, you should be given the opportunity to talk with someone about all the options so that you can come to an informed decision.

## Chromosomal abnormalities

Every healthy baby carries 23 chromosomes from mum, and the same number from dad. This is what determines whether it'll have Auntie Nora's nose or dad's eyes. Sometimes, though, this doesn't work out and up to half of all miscarriages are due to chromosomal abnormalities. It's important to remember that this is nature's way of getting rid of a mistake, and is nobody's fault. On occasion the pregnancy doesn't end, and so the foetus continues to develop despite having problems. There may be too many or too few chromosomes (aneuploidy), or some of them can be damaged or put together in the wrong order.

## Down's syndrome

Down's syndrome means the baby has 3 chromosome 21's instead of 2 (one from each parent remember). This problem is also called trisomy 21. Ultrasound markers may be visible, but there will usually be physical defects too. So if your anomaly scan does show markers, a careful examination of the baby will be carried out to see if there are any other signs of abnormality.

Other chromosomal problems include Edward's syndrome (trisomy 18) and Patau's syndrome (trisomy 13).

Most people are aware that older mums have a higher risk of having a baby with chromosomal abnormalities: if you are 35 years old or more, this is something to be taken into consideration.

| Maternal age | Chance of Down's syndrome | |
| :---: | :---: | :---: |
| | At 12 weeks | At birth |
| 20 | 1 in 1070 | 1 in 1530 |
| 25 | 950 | 1350 |
| 30 | 630 | 900 |
| 32 | 460 | 660 |
| 34 | 310 | 450 |
| 35 | 250 | 360 |
| 36 | 200 | 280 |
| 38 | 120 | 170 |
| 40 | 70 | 100 |
| 42 | 40 | 55 |
| 44 | 20 | 30 |

The likelihood of spontaneous miscarriage with a Down's syndrome foetus between 12 – 40 weeks is 40%. Between 16 – 40 weeks it's 20%. For trisomies 18 and 13 between 12 – 40 weeks it's 80%.

The risk of a subsequent pregnancy having chromosomal abnormalities at 12 weeks: at age 25 it's 1 in 117 (up from 1 in 946 for a woman with a previous normal pregnancy). For age 35 it's 1 in 87 (up from 1 in 249). This represents a 0.75% higher risk.

## Contraindications

Is ultrasound safe? In general, yes. There is no significant evidence that it causes harm to the foetus. Ultrasound is used therapeutically because of its ability to heat internal tissues at high frequencies; obstetric transducers are not used for this. However, some studies have found a possible link to low birthweight, left handedness and slightly slower development in speech.

A 1979-81 study done in Norway on 2161 children concluded that there was a possible association between routine ultrasonography and the child's non right handedness, but found no other correlations ie neurological problems. Speaking as a southpaw myself I'd just like to say that I don't see this is a problem, although if you're worried about your child's ability to use a tin opener you may feel differently. **(1)**

The same researchers re-evaluated the children involved at age 9 – 19 and found no difference in their ability to read and write compared to other children.

An Australian study looked at whether the number of tests made any difference, using a group of 1415 women who had 5 ultrasound scans at different stages of their pregnancies (the intensive group). A control group of 1419 only had 1 scan. There was "significantly higher intrauterine growth restriction" in the intensive group. The conclusion of the researchers was that this may have been due to chance, but it would be prudent for scans to be repeated only on women who needed them. **(2)**

A follow up study was done by the same researchers on the children born of the intensively scanned mothers, at 1 year old and 8 years respectively. Speech, language, neurological development and behaviour were examined, and the children were found to have no significant difference to other children. **(3)**

## Doppler ultrasound scans

Doppler scans are used to check foetal cardiac health later in the pregnancy. They do this by detecting pulsations in the baby's heart and blood vessels, notably the umbilical artery, aorta, middle cerebral arteries and uterine arcuate arteries. Reduced blood flow can be a sign of problems such as congenital heart abnormalities.

Doppler scans can be useful in predicting pre eclampsia, and have been found to be instrumental in reducing perinatal deaths connected to maternal hypertension or reduced foetal growth, but they are not part of the normal array of prenatal tests in the UK. Because they use a higher frequency of sound, there have been some concerns as to their effect on the foetus, though there is little evidence as yet one way or the other. In particular, pulsed doppler can produce heating effects in body tissues.

A study reported in the Cochrane Database of Systematic Reviews looked at several pieces of research on doppler scans, and whether they had any benefits when used routinely. The 5 trials examined (the latest one in 1999) involved 14,338 women. The authors concluded that, for low-risk pregnancies, there was no benefit to the routine use of doppler scanning, and there may be a small risk of harm. For high-risk pregnancies however, it can be useful in detecting foetal problems. **(4)**

Another study looking at foetal heart rate as a possible diagnostic aid examined the evidence that foetuses with chromosomal abnormalities show either slower or faster heart rates than normal ones. Blood flow in the ductus venosus was measured at 11 – 14 weeks using doppler ultrasound. Absent or reversed flow during heart contraction was found in 57 of 63 chromosomally abnormal foetuses (90.5%) as opposed to 13 of 423 normal foetuses (3.1%). However in 7 of the 13 a later scan at 14 – 16 weeks demonstrated a major cardiac defect. The study's authors concluded that although it was not practical to make ductal flow examination part of routine screening, it could be very useful as a secondary screening method. This would achieve a major reduction in the rate of primary screening false positives, and thus of women going forward to have CVS and amniocentesis. The overall need for these invasive tests could be reduced from 5% to less than 0.5%. **(5)**

### Doppler for hire

Doppler units can be hired or bought from various companies, so you can listen to your baby's heartbeat at home. There has not been any scientific research (that I could find) as to whether listening to your baby several times a day, or even once daily for a week, is safe.

## Useful websites/references

**http://www.fetalmedicine.com**
Site of the Fetal Medicine Centre based in Harley St, London

**www.babycentre.co.uk**
**www.nelh.nhs.uk/screening**
UK National Screening Committee

**http://www.rcog.org.uk**
Royal College of Obstetricians and Gynaecologists (RCOG)

## Other references

1 Routine ultrasonography in utero and subsequent handedness and neurological development
Salvesen KA; Vatten LJ; Eik-Nes SH; Hugdahl K; Bakketeig LS
Department of Gynaecology and Obstetrics, University Medical Centre, Trondheim, Norway.
BMJ, 1993 Jul 17, 307:6897, 159-64

2 Effects of frequent ultrasound during pregnancy: a randomised controlled trial
Authors: Newnham JP; Evans SF; Michael CA; Stanley FJ; Landau LI

University Department of Obstetrics and Gynaecology, King Edward Memorial Hospital, Subiaco, Perth, Western Australia.
Lancet, 1993 Oct 9, 342:8876, 887-91

**3** The Lancet 2004; 364:2038-2044
DOI:10.1016/S0140-6736(04)17516-8
Effects of repeated prenatal ultrasound examinations on childhood outcome up to 8 years of age: follow-up of a randomised controlled trial
John P Newnham a,  Dorota A Doherty a,  Garth E Kendall b,  Stephen R Zubrick c,  Louis L Landau d  Fiona J Stanley b

a. School of Women's and Infants' Health, The University of Western Australia at King Edward Memorial Hospital, Subiaco, Western Australia 6008
b. TVW Telethon Institute for Child Health Research
c. Curtin Centre for Developmental Health, Institute for Child Health Research
d. Faculty of Medicine and Dentistry, The University of Western Australia, Perth, Western Australia

School of Women's and Infants' Health, King Edward Memorial Hospital, Subiaco, Perth, Western Australia

**4** Routine Doppler ultrasound in pregnancy does not have health benefits for women or babies, and may do some harm.
The Cochrane Database of Systematic Reviews 2006 Issue 1
Copyright © 2006 The Cochrane Collaboration. Published by John Wiley & Sons, Ltd.
Routine Doppler ultrasound in pregnancy
Bricker L, Neilson JP

**5 http://www.fetalmedicine.com**
The 11-13 (+6day) week scan. KH Nicolaides, NJ Sebire, RJM Snijders

# 11 Amniocentesis

This is a diagnostic test recommended if you have had a screening test (ie ultrasound) that has indicated there may be a problem with your baby. It involves a needle being inserted into the uterus, under ultrasound guidance, to take a sample of amniotic fluid. Usually it's done between 16-18 weeks. The fluid contains cells from the baby, and these are cultured (grown) in a laboratory so that karyotyping (genetic testing) can be done.

The sensation of the needle going in and passing through the uterine muscle is described as "discomfort" – mostly by men. Female consensus seems to be that it's mildly painful but bearable. Following the procedure you may experience cramping, slight vaginal bleeding, or a small amount of leakage of amniotic fluid from the vagina. Sometimes the cells don't grow in the lab, so more have to be taken, but this doesn't happen very often. However, the more times you have amniocentesis, the higher the risk of miscarriage.

The most usual reason why you might have amniocentesis is because previous scans have shown a possibility of chromosomal abnormalities, such as Down's syndrome (trisomy 21), or there may be a family genetic trait like cystic fibrosis or sickle cell anaemia. The amniotic fluid itself can also be tested for the presence of alphafoetoprotein (AFP), high levels of which indicates that the foetus has spina bifida – this has a 95% accuracy rate.

There is a 1 in 100 to 1 in 300 risk of miscarriage with amniocentesis. However amniocentesis should only be suggested if there has already been an indication that there may be a problem. In a normal pregnancy it is not necessary. Results can take 3 or 4 weeks, which is a long time to wait when you're worried. Around 15,000 women a year have the test. False positive rate is low: around 1 in 1000.

## Complications

Membrane rupture, causing leakage of amniotic fluid, happens more often in women who have had amniocentesis. The leakage is usually small and stops within a week.

There may be a risk that if the mother has an infection such as HIV or toxoplasmosis, this can be transmitted to the baby. The amniotic fluid itself can become infected, leading to miscarriage, but this is very rare, occurring in around 1 in 1000 procedures. It's also possible that the baby has a slightly higher risk of clubfoot, hip dislocation and respiratory problems.

Research has shown that early amniocentesis (10-13 weeks) carries increased risk of foetal death, talipes equinovarus (rocker bottom feet), failed culture growth requiring a repeat test, and post procedural amniotic fluid leakage. The conclusion of these studies was that amniocentesis should not be performed before 13 weeks.

## New screening protocols

In 2004 the UK National Screening Committee (UKNSC) recommended that new screening programmes for Down's syndrome don't need to include karyotyping (the method used traditionally) and can offer prenatal diagnosis for DS with FISH (fluorescence in-situ hybridisation) or PCR (polymerase chain reaction, which is a quick way of copying little bits of DNA for genetic testing) as rapid aneuploidy testing. The UKNSC also recommended that FISH or PCR tests should only include trisomies 13, 18, and 21.

This recommendation is controversial because FISH and PCR are considered by many to be less accurate than karyotyping, but are cheaper and quicker to do. An assessment study was carried out by Caine and Maltby et al of the UK Association of Clinical Cytogeneticists (ACC). 23 prenatal cytogenetic labs in the UK – they analyse cells taken using CVS or amniocentesis – submitted data between 1999 and 2004. These data included details of all abnormal karyotypes by 'reason for referral' and assessed the efficiency of FISH and PCR rapid tests in detecting chromosomal abnormalities.

Of 119,528 amniotic fluid (AV) samples, and 23,077 chorionic villus (CV) samples, rapid aneuploidy testing would have resulted in 1 in 100 and 1 in 40 positives respectively being missed. Of these missed positives, 293 (30%) of 1006 AF samples and 152 (45%) of CV samples showed a substantial risk of abnormal outcome. Out of 34,995 AF samples and 3049 CV samples that were subject to both karyotyping and rapid testing, the best results were obtained when karyotyping and either FISH or PCR were used together. The study concluded that replacing karyotyping with rapid testing (after a positive screening test for Down's syndrome) will result in substantial numbers of babies being born "with hitherto preventable mental or physical handicaps, and represents a substantial change in the outcome quality of prenatal testing offered to couples in the UK."

In a later comment the authors say: "The fundamental difference between these two approaches is that with karyotyping, the information can be considered by the patients and their clinicians and an informed choice made on the basis of the evidence, whereas with rapid aneuploidy testing this choice is withdrawn. We believe that this strategy could be severely detrimental for up to 100 neonates per year in the UK.

"We believe that antenatal karyotyping must be retained, but with turnaround times near the 7 days achieved by some UK laboratories. Furthermore, we believe that it is ironic in an era of "patient empowerment" that the UKNSC is adopting a paternalistic approach to determining what patients should or should not know after prenatal testing." **(1)**

# Useful websites/references

**http://www.guysandstthomas.nhs.uk**
pdf of leaflet: The Amniocentesis Test: Some General Information. 2002
Also available as hardcopy

**http://patients.uptodate.com**
UpToDate performs a continuous review of over 350 journals and other resources.

**http://www.medic8.com**
A-Z Health Information site

# Other references

1  Lancet 2005 July 9-15;366(9480):123-8
   Prenatal detection of Down's syndrome by rapid aneuploidy testing for chromo-
   somes 13, 18, and 21 by FISH or PCR without a full karyotype: a cytogenetic risk
   assessment.
   Caine A, Maltby AE, Parkin CA, Waters JJ, Crolla JA; UK Association of Clinical
   Cytogeneticists (ACC).
   Regional Cytogenetics Unit, St James' University Hospital, Leeds, UK.

# 12  Chorionic villus sampling

Chorionic Villi are what your placenta is made of, and they have the same chromosomes as your baby. Chorionic Villus Sampling (CVS) consists of taking a small sample from the placenta and doing a DNA test for signs of chromosomal abnormalities such as Down's syndrome, Tay Sachs and cystic fibrosis. This test can also discover the sex of your baby, and is usually done at 10 to 12 weeks of gestation. Results shouldn't take more than a few days.

A woman may consider having CVS if:
- She is 35 years or older
- She has had an abnormal screening test result
- She has previous pregnancy history of a genetic disorder, or
- She has a close relative who has

There are 2 methods of taking a CVS: transcervical and transabdominal. The first (TC CVS) involves a cannula (thin tube) being passed through the cervix into the placenta where it collects a small sample of tissue. This is carried out under ultrasound guidance.

The second method, TA CVS, requires a needle going through the abdomen into the placenta, being careful to avoid puncturing the amniotic sac. The needle collects the sample and withdraws. Ultrasound guidance is required for accurate placing of the needle.

Both these methods are usually successful at the first attempt; it is sometimes necessary to repeat the process if an inadequate amount of tissue was collected.

## Contraindications

There are certain circumstances in which transcervical CVS is not appropriate. These include cervical stenosis, where the opening of the cervix is constricted; cervical or lower uterine myomas, which are benign muscle tumours; cervical infection; and severe bending of the uterus making it difficult to manoeuvre the cannula.

Contraindications (reasons why it's not a good idea to do something) for transabdominal CVS include extreme bending of the uterus where there could be part of the intestine between the uterus and the abdominal wall – this could be punctured by the needle; and the foetus positioned so as to block access to the placenta.

## Complications

The most serious complications from CVS are damage to the foetus, and miscarriage. CVS is not known to affect the risk of stillbirth or infant death. On average, CVS is associated with a 2.4% higher than normal miscarriage rate. The TC CVS procedure has, however, in some studies shown an 11% higher risk, compared to 6% for the TA CVS (this last is on a par with the risk associated with amniocentesis). The risk of miscarriage is also higher if the foetus is small for gestational age, and if the test is done 3 or more times. There is also the significant variable of the operator's skill and experience.

Four randomised studies that looked at the rate of miscarriage following 1st trimester CVS compared the rates to that of amniocentesis done at 16 weeks. Around 10,000 pregnancies were included, and results showed that where the tests were carried out in centres with experienced staff, miscarriage rates for both CVS and amniocentesis were similar. This study concluded that the higher rate of miscarriage for CVS reported elsewhere was connected to operator inexperience.

The CVS test may in certain circumstances have a slightly higher risk of miscarriage than amniocentesis, but is done earlier in the pregnancy so can give you more time to make a decision if you get a significant result. There's a possibility that the test gives a false positive result (ie suggests a chromosome abnormality exists when in fact it doesn't) in a small number of instances, possibly 1 in 100. If there is doubt, an amniocentesis test may be necessary to clarify things. The chances of CVS giving a false negative (showing no chromosomal abnormality when in fact there is one) is about 1 in 1000.

In the early 1990s severe limb abnormalities were reported in 5 of 289 pregnancies that had undergone CVS at less than 10 weeks gestation. Other reports confirmed this association, and analysis of 75 cases showed a definite connection between the severity of the deformity and gestational age at time of sampling. Background incidence (normal occurrence) of serious limb defects is around 1.8 per 10,000 live births. Following early CVS this figure is estimated to increase to 1 in 200-1000 cases. For this reason, it is recommended by the Fetal Medical Foundation (a UK charity) that CVS is not done before 11 weeks.

Up to a third of women who have had CVS report vaginal spotting ie slight bleeding. Heavier bleeding occurs in less than 6% and is more common after TC CVS, which also may also have a higher risk of infection.

There is a chance that CVS can cause small amounts of foetal blood to be released into the mother's circulation (foetomaternal haemorrhage). In mothers who are Rh- (rhesus negative) this may trigger an immune response. Such mothers should receive Rhogam (RhD immune globulin) after CVS to prevent this.

If there is a risk of sickle cell anaemia, CVS can also be used to test for which type of haemoglobin the baby has. Cells collected via CVS are examined for the presence of the sickle cell gene.

## Confined placental mosaicism

This is a rare situation in which the placenta shows abnormal cells that are not present in the foetus. In such a case, an amniocentesis would be necessary to confirm the result.

# Useful websites/references

**www.patients.uptodate.com**
Patient Information: Chorionic Villus Sampling. Alessandro Ghidini MD, Rodney McLaren MD

**http://www.sicklecellsociety.org**
The charity for sickle cell anaemia

**www.fetalmedicine.com**
Site of the Fetal Medicine Centre based in Harley St, London

**http://www.medic8.com**
A-Z Health Information site

**www.nelh.nhs.uk/screening**
UK National Screening Committee

# 13 Nuchal translucency

This is an ultrasound test that looks at the back of the baby's neck where fluid collects. The translucency (how light passes through) is checked because increased nuchal translucency (NT) can mean that the baby is likely to have Down's syndrome (trisomy 21). It's a screening test, so is used to estimate the risk of Down's syndrome – it cannot provide a diagnosis, which is why, if risk is present, you will be advised to have a CVS or amniocentesis.

An NT scan is usually done from 11-13 weeks. Before this the baby is too small to be examined properly, and after this the excess fluid that the test measures may be reabsorbed by the baby's lymphatic system. Sometimes if the baby is positioned awkwardly it's necessary to do a vaginal scan instead, which gives clearer images.

The sonographer measures the crown rump length (CRL) to confirm the age of the pregnancy, then measures the width of the NT. You'll be able to see your baby's head, spine, hands and feet at this stage. As well as Down's syndrome, some other major abnormalities may be ruled out by this scan, but you'll still be advised to have the anomaly scan at 20 weeks to check for other problems.

What's a normal NT measurement? At around 11 weeks, up to 2.00mm is usual. By 14 weeks it will be around 2.8mm. Even if NT is more than this it doesn't necessarily mean there's a problem – normal babies can have increased fluid too. 9 out of 10 babies with an NT of between 2.5mm and 3.5mm will be fine. Remember this is a screening test, not a diagnostic test: it may show increased risk, but that risk needs to be confirmed by a more detailed test such as CVS or amniocentesis.

The NT scan has an accuracy of around 75%, with a false positive rate of less than 5%. Your risk of having a chromosomally abnormal baby is assessed by combining the background risk (normal occurrence) with your own personal risk based on the scan, your age, and any other significant criteria.

Because sonographers have to be specially trained, and there's a nationwide shortage of them, not all hospitals provide NT scans, so you will need to check if yours does. If not, the test can be done privately.

## Useful websites/references

**www.nelh.nhs.uk/screening**
UK National Screening Committee

**Down's Syndrome Association**
The charity for Down's syndrome

# 14  Other tests

There is a battery of private tests you can pay for.

Blood test: checks levels of hCG (human chorionic gonadotropin) and PAPP-A (pregnancy associated plasma protein). Accuracy up to 60%.

The Combined test is NT and blood test. Acc. up to 90%.

In the 2nd trimester, from 15 to 20 weeks:
- Double test: hCG and AFP (alpha fetoprotein) Acc: 59%
- Triple test: hCG, AFP plus uE3 (unconjugated oestriol)
- Quadruple test: hCG, AFP, uE3 plus Inhibin A. Acc: 75%

Integrated test: NT and PAPP-A in 1st trimester with the quadruple in the 2nd. Accuracy up to 94% for Down's syndrome.

Serum integrated test: blood test for PAPP-A in 1st trimester with the quadruple in the 2nd.

OSCAR is "One stop clinic for the assessment of risk" using a fairly new technique (random access immunoassay analyzer using time-resolved-amplified-cryptate-emission, since you ask). This enables testing to be automated, accurate and reproducible within 30 minutes of obtaining a blood sample. Various hospitals provide it and it will cost you around £100. It involves an NT scan and the double blood test (hCG and PAPP-A) to test for Down's syndrome, done at the same time. The accuracy rate is 90%.

Given that people with Down's syndrome have very small and/or flat noses, a recent test might seem to be blindingly obvious in a "why did nobody think of this before" sort of way. Quite simply, seeing your baby's nasal bone on a scan means it is very unlikely to have Down's. When this is added to the OSCAR tests, accuracy increases up to 97%. See, it's not all rocket science.

Some hospitals offer an NT scan to everyone at 11-14 weeks, some a blood test for Down's syndrome at 16 weeks, some only offer ladies of a certain age a test for Downs – and some don't offer you any screening tests at all. If you go private you can expect to pay anywhere from £100 - £450 depending on which test you're having. But even at that, it's probably cheaper than a trip to the dentist.

So if you're having a normal, healthy pregnancy, it may be worth considering whether you need (or want to pay for) a battery of tests. What do those nice people at NICE have to say about all this? They have produced a helpful leaflet which is available online (pdf), or as a hardcopy. They recommend that you have the 2 basic ultrasound screening tests: 10-13 weeks, and 18-20. If you are having a normal pregnancy you should not need any more than this.

Screening tests for Down's syndrome should have an accuracy rate of no less than 60%, with a false positive rate of no more than 5%. The following tests are approved:

- 11 to 14 weeks: NT, combined test (ultrasound & blood test)
- 14 to 20 weeks: Triple test, quadruple test
- 11-14 and 13-18 weeks: Integrated test, serum integrated test

By April 2007 all women should be offered screening tests for Down's syndrome with an accuracy rate of over 75% and a false positive rate of less than 3%. The tests that meet this standard are:

- 11 to 14 weeks: combined test
- 14 to 20 weeks: quadruple test
- 11-14 and 14-20 weeks: serum integrated test.

## Useful websites/references

http://www.babycentre.co.uk
http://www.fetalmedicine.com
The 11 – 13 (+6day) week scan

KH Nicolaides, NJ Sebire, RJM Snijders (A huge and exhaustive piece of research)
http://www.nice.org.uk

# Other references

Prenatal Diagnosis 2005 Feb;25(2): 133-6
Re-evaluation of risk for Down syndrome by means of the combined test in pregnant women of 35 years or more.
Centini G, Rosignoli L, Scarinci R, Faldini E, Morra C, Centini G, Petraglia F.
Prenatal Diagnosis Centre, Chair of Obstetrics and Gynecology, Department of Pediatrics, Obstetrics, and Reproductive Medicine, University of Siena, Siena Italy.

Ginekologia Polska 2004 Mar;75(3):197-202

Combination of screening tests for fetal abnormalities in the first and second pregnancy trimesters
[Article in Polish]
Sieroszewski P, Suzin J, Bas-Budecka E.
Instytut Ginekologii i Poloznictwa Uniwersytetu Medycznego w Lodzi.

Pubmed: Beijing Da Xue Xue Bao. 2006 Feb 18;38(1):49-52

Chromosomal abnormalities and adverse pregnancy outcome with maternal serum second trimester triple screening test for fetal Down syndrome in 4860 Chinese women.
Xia YP, Zhu MW, Li XT, Zhou HP, Wang J, Lv JX, Zhong N.
The Hospital of Obstetrics and Gynecology, Fudan University, Shanghai 200011, China.

Routine antenatal care for healthy pregnant women (leaflet)

NO310 1P 20K Oct 03 (ABA) nice.org.uk (pdf)

# Part 2
# Labour

## 15  Home birth

In Britain, at the beginning of the 20th century, 99% of babies were born at home. Since then, hospital has become the preferred option, partly because birth has become medicalised, and by the 1980s the home birth rate was less than 1%. By the end of the 90s the rate had crept up to 2.2%, but access to a home birth service can vary from area to area, and women are not always encouraged to think of it as an option.

### Is it safe?

The definitive scientific study done on home birth is the National Birthday Trust - Report of the Confidential Enquiry into Home Births. This is probably the most comprehensive study of home birth ever undertaken in the UK. Its intention was to include all women who booked a home birth in the UK in 1994. This involved 5971 low-risk women who were matched like for like. That is, women who were booked for home birth at 37 weeks gestation were matched with hospital booked mothers who were also low risk, and similar in terms of age, health, number of previous births, past obstetric history, and where they lived.

Note that these are *planned* home births or *planned* hospital deliveries. Some previous studies have included in the home birth statistics all births not delivered in hospital, including unexpected prematures, hidden or secret births (such as pregnant teenagers who didn't tell anyone), unbooked births, and other high-risk cases, thus skewing the results against the safety of home birth.

84% of the mothers had given birth before, 16% were first timers. Those who had had a previous Caesarean were at 1% for the home birth group, and 3% for the hospital group. Planning a home birth reduced by 50% the chances of women having assisted or Caesarean births. The overall rate of these events was very low, because mainly only low-risk women booked for a home birth.

Home births, including transfers, were less likely to involve post-partum haemorrhage. Home birth mothers had fewer episiotomies but more first-degree perineal tears. Second-degree tears occurred at the same rate in both groups. All cervical tears occurred in the hospital group.

Of the women in planned home birth who'd had a previous child, 9.7% had previous assisted deliveries and 1.4% had had Caesareans. The rate of transfer from home to hospital among the previously assisted group was 15.6%, and among the previous Caesareans 28% - in other words 72% had a home VBAC (vaginal birth after Caesarean) without any problems. The overall percentage of transferred mothers who had a Caesarean was 11.2%.

## Overall outcomes

|  | Planned home births (including transfers) | Planned hospital births |
|---|---|---|
| Spontaneous vaginal delivery | 94.7% | 90.2% |
| Assisted (forceps, ventouse) | 2.4% | 5.4% |
| Caesarean | 2.0% | 4.1% |

# Planned home births: transfer rate

The total number of women who were transferred was 769, all of whom had a healthy baby except for 2 stillbirths and 2 neonatal deaths. 16% were transferred to hospital. 60% of first time mums delivered at home and 40% were transferred. 90% of previous-birth mothers had their babies at home, and only 10% were transferred.

The main reason for transfer was slow or no progress, at 37.2%. 24.8% were due to premature rupture of membranes (mostly before start of labour), and foetal distress prompted 14.8%, with 1 cord prolapse.

As women are transferred from home to hospital only if there is a problem, this is the highest risk group. It is likely that had these births been planned for hospital instead of home, the results would have been the same.

# Pain relief

Home birth mothers were much less likely to use drugs for pain relief compared to women in hospital. The following table gives the results as reported by midwives; a lot of mothers used more than one method of pain relief, hence the totals add up to more than 100.

| Pain Relief | Planned home overall | Planned hospital | Home births (born at home) | Transfers from home to hospital |
|---|---|---|---|---|
| DRUGS | | | | |
| Entonox | 52.6% | 72.1% | 50.1% | 65.8% |
| Pethidine/ Demerol | 7.5% | 30.3% | 4.3% | 23.7% |
| Epidural | 2.8% (all transfers) | 11.3% | 0 | 17.9% |
| Spinal Block | 0.7% | 1.3% | 0 | 4.1% |

NON-DRUG METHODS

| | | | | |
|---|---|---|---|---|
| Relaxation | 49.0% | 30.1% | 50.3% | 43.1% |
| TENS | 22% | 15.4% | 20.6% | 28.8% |
| Warm water | 24.4% | 8% | 24.5% | 24% |
| Aromatherapy | 5.2% | 0.9% | 5.2% | 5.1% |
| Homeopathy | 3.4% | 0.3% | 3.3% | 4% |
| Acupuncture | 0.6% | 0 | 0.5% | 0.9% |
| None | 17.1% | 8.6% | 18.8% | 7.9% |

*Chart from Homebirth.org website*

Home born babies had fewer interventions: 11.3% were suctioned (planned hospital 18%), bag and mask 5.6% (PH 9.1%), intubation 0.6% (PH 0.8%).

Out of 5971 planned home births there were 5 stillbirth/neonatal deaths, and also 5 of the 4724 planned hospital births. The national rate was 8 per 1000 births. The study concluded that these figures were too low to provide a meaningful comparison.

The evidence-based maternity care bible, A Guide to Effective Care in Pregnancy and Childbirth, states:

"Several methodologically sound observational studies have compared the outcomes of planned home births (irrespective of the eventual place of birth) with planned hospital births for women with similar characteristics. A meta-analysis of these studies showed no maternal mortality and no statistically significant differences in perinatal mortality between the groups. The number of births included in the studies was sufficiently large to rule out any major difference in perinatal mortality risk in either direction."

In 1993 a government report called Changing Childbirth concluded that there was no evidence that a hospital birth was safer than a home birth for healthy women, and women should be given the choice which option they would prefer. This concludes that home birth is perfectly safe for low-risk mothers.

You'll have noticed that 'low risk' mothers are referred to a lot – most authorities use this phrase out of caution. Pregnancies defined as 'high risk' include multiple births, first time births, older mothers, and mothers who may have, for example, diabetes, high blood pressure and heart disease. Again, you are hearing the voice of caution, so if you feel strongly about having a home birth and you have been classified as high risk, ask why.

An oft-quoted study called "Place of birth and perinatal mortality" using data from a British national survey of 1970 found that in all except the 'very high risk' categories, home birth was safer than hospital birth. The hospital PMR (perinatal mortality rate) was 27.8 per 1000 births, as opposed to 5.4 per 1000 home births. In fact, the PMR for high risk home births was 15.5 per 1000, lower than the hospital low risk PMR rate of 17.9 per 1000. [1]

And the 1992 House of Commons Select Committee on Maternity Services, now known as the Winterton report, making more than 100 recommendations and conclusions on pregnancy, labour and postnatal care, said "On the basis of what we have heard, this Committee must draw the conclusion that the policy of encouraging all women to give birth in hospitals cannot be justified on grounds of safety."

## Your choice

In 1995 The Royal College of General Practitioners and the Royal College of Midwives issued a joint statement declaring:

"Women wishing to arrange a home birth should be able to do so. General practitioners who do not wish to provide care for home births should refer women to a local midwife or the local supervisor of midwives (or to a general practitioner who does provide full maternity care)."

You can also write to the manager of your local community midwifery services to say you want a home birth. Or you can go for the independent midwife option. An IM can carry out antenatal care, attend the birth, and provide postnatal care too. Costs vary according to where you live and which services you opt for, but in general you'll be looking to pay £1500 - £4000. Bear in mind that, if you do choose a home birth, you can change your mind right up to the last minute and go for a hospital transfer.

## Useful websites/references

1 Journal of the Royal College of General Practitioners 1985;35(277):390-394
Place of birth and perinatal mortality, M Tew

**http://www.homebirth.org.uk**
Excellent site under auspices of National Childbirth Trust.

**http://www.babycentre.co.uk**
**http://www.activebirthcentre.com**
Encourages women's empowerment in labour
**http://bmj.bmjjournals.com/cgi/content/full/313/7068/1276**
British Medical Journal Editorial, 23 November 1996
BMJ 1996;313:1276-1277 (23 November)
Editorials Home birth: Safe in selected women, and with adequate infrastructure and support

**http://www.aims.org.uk**
Association for Improvement in Maternity Services

**http://www.birthchoiceuk.com**
Information on maternity units, statistics etc

**http://www.independentmidwives.org.uk/**
Fully qualified self employed midwives who have chosen to work outside the NHS in order to practice the midwife's role to its fullest extent.

**http://www.babyworld.co.uk**
This site very useful for regional and local health authority stats.

**http://www.nctpregnancyandbabycare.com**
National Childcare Trust

# Other references

Obstetric Myths versus Research Realities. Henci Goer. Bergin & Garvey 1995. ISBN: 0897894278. Every mother-to-be should read this!

A Guide to Effective Care in Pregnancy and Childbirth, Murray Enkin et al, Oxford University Press Inc (USA), 2000. ISBN: 019263173X.

Practical Midwife 1999 Jul-Aug;2(7):35-9
Birth at home.
Chamberlain G, Wraight A, Crowley P.
Obstetrics at Singleton Hospital, Swansea.

# 16  Induction

You've set the date, you've organised the catering, you've sent out the invitations, but the star guest is nowhere in sight. Pregnancy generally takes between 39 and 41 weeks, but sometimes it seems it will never end. There are sound medical reasons for inducing labour, ie pre-eclampsia, but here we're looking at late arrivals of a non-medical nature.

According to Naegele's Rule, the due date is 280 days from the first day of the last period. But we aren't all as regular as we'd like, and this way of doing the sums can sometimes mean that your EDD (Estimated Delivery Date) is earlier than it should be. Ultrasound scans are an accurate means of estimating DD, and recent thinking suggests that if Naegele's Rule is applied using 283 days instead, it's as accurate as the ultrasound scan-based method.

## Induction rates

There is also the question of whether the hospital has a policy of induction past a certain date: for some hospitals the induction rate is as high as 25%, for others it's as low as 14%, regardless of whether they specialise in high-risk pregnancies. In England the national rate is 20.55%, or slightly more than one in every five women. The Midwives Research and Information Service says:

"Where women opt for expectant management (in other words 'wait and see') they can be reassured that it is highly probable that they will labour spontaneously (without needing an induction) before 42 completed weeks and that the likelihood of stillbirth remains very low".

So why can't you just sit there, getting more huge by the day, and wait for nature to take its course? Induction is considered necessary after a certain time because of the risk of stillbirth. This is about 1 in 3000 at 37 weeks, increasing to 3 in 3000 at 42 and 6 in 3000 at

43. These are very low numbers, and it's still not clear whether babies die because the pregnancy has gone on for longer than it should, or because there was a problem which caused the pregnancy to become extended.

Generally, health professionals give you up to 10 days beyond the due date before getting out the spanners, but sometimes induction doesn't work, in which case you will need to consider whether to wait a bit longer, or go for a Caesarean.

Labour can be induced in a number of ways:

1   A membrane sweep, in which the membranes surrounding your baby are separated from the cervix. It also causes the release of prostaglandins which will in most cases induce labour.

2   Breaking the waters, known as ARM. Not the insertion of a limb into your nether regions, this is Artificially Rupturing the Membranes, whereby the doctor passes a long thin probe through the cervix to make a small break in the membranes. 70% of mothers give birth within 24 hours, and 90% within 72 hours of their waters breaking.

3   Inserting a gel or pessary containing prostaglandin into the vagina to ripen, or soften, the cervix. Prostaglandin is a hormone-like substance and enables uterine contractions to begin.

If one of the above methods is tried and found to be ineffective, intravenous administration of the hormone oxytocin – in a synthetic form called Syntocinon – can be given. This triggers contractions and the dose can be adjusted to produce an appropriate rate of contraction. A combination of these methods can be used, according to your particular circumstances.

There are other, gentler and less invasive methods you can try too: making love for example. Sexual orgasm releases oxytocin (see above) and semen contains prostaglandin. If your waters have broken, intercourse is inadvisable as this can lead to infection. Nipple stimulation (whoopee) releases oxytocin too, and can help with the ripening of the cervix, or promote contractions. Walking may help because gravity presses the baby's head against the cervix, again releasing oxytocin. It can also persuade baby to "drop" into a better position which may help trigger the birth process.

Because it isn't an immediate or urgent event, you should always be given time to think about an induction, so that you can make your own decision whether to wait for a couple of days (and have lots of sex and nipple tweaking), or go for the intervention.

Induction puts you into the second stage of labour, and as the first stage is the one that prompts your body to produce its natural pain relief, you may find yourself experiencing serious pain rather suddenly. Fond plans of a drug free birth may fly out the window at this point, and if you do feel you're trying to give birth to an elephant don't be ashamed to ask for pain control ("I want the f**king drugs and I want them NOW!")

## What are the risks?

Induction may not work immediately; sometimes repeat treatments are necessary and you may not go into actual labour for several days. ARM isn't always effective, and because your waters are broken, you will need to be watched in case of infection. If syntocinon is given, it can cause strong contractions which may put the baby under stress, and there is a very small risk that your uterus can be overstimulated, which reduces the oxygen supply to the baby, so you will need to be attached to an Electronic Foetal Monitor. This records your contractions and the baby's heart beat. High doses of syntocinon can overstimulate the uterus, causing it to tear. It may also lead to irregular maternal heartbeat, post partum bleeding, and has been known to cause jaundice in newborns.

# Useful websites/references

**http://www.babycentre.co.uk**
**http://www.babyworld.co.uk**
This site very useful for regional and local health authority stats.

**http://www.nctpregnancyandbabycare.com**
National Childcare Trust

**http://www.dh.gov.uk**
Dept of Health site. The Pregnancy Book March 2005 edition
Pdf or browsable, hardcopy. Dept of Health, 31/3/2005. 266528. 152p.

**http://www.marchofdimes.com**
**http://www.rcog.org.uk**
Royal College of Obstetricians and Gynaecologists (RCOG)

# 17  Assisted delivery

You are more likely to require this following an induction or previous Caesarean birth.

Forceps are like a pair of large salad tongs, made of stainless steel, which are curved to fit a baby's head. The doctor will pull as you push, drawing the baby down the birth canal. After a forceps delivery you may feel sore and bruised, experience difficulty in urinating, and may leak urine unexpectedly. It can also make you constipated. There is some risk of permanent bladder or rectal damage, and faecal incontinence. The baby may have bruising for a few days, and the facial nerve can be damaged, causing the mouth to droop on one side – a palsy – but this is usually temporary.

Ventouse delivery (vacuum extraction) is preferred over forceps as it is safer and has fewer side effects. The ventouse cup – either silicone or metal – is placed on the baby's head inside you, and the air drawn out using a vacuum pump. As with forceps, the doctor pulls while you push. Afterwards, your baby may resemble a conehead, but this won't last, and nor will the cephalhaematoma (blood blister) that sometimes occurs on the scalp.

## Useful websites/references

http://www.babycentre.co.uk
http://www.marchofdimes.com
http://www.rcog.org.uk
Royal College of Obstetricians and Gynaecologists (RCOG)

# 18  Caesarean section

You may not have much choice as to whether or not you have a Caesarean, because it's usually prompted by factors such as a problematic birth or the safety of your baby. But Caesarean rates do vary between hospitals and it's worth checking these out. Some hospital Caesarean rates are around 13% of births while others are as high as 30%. This may be because health professionals have different ideas as to what constitutes an emergency; some are more cautious than others. The rates are rising, and one of the reasons for this is that more women are requesting a Caesarean over 42 weeks.

Reasons for a planned Caesarean include: breech birth, multiple birth, previous invasive uterine surgery including several Caesareans, placental problems such as placenta praevia (placenta planted so low in the uterus as to cause an obstruction), abruptio placenta where the placenta becomes detached from the uterine wall, or risk of the baby contracting an infection such as genital herpes while moving through the vagina.

Unplanned Caesarean can result from the following: the baby develops an irregular heartbeat and may not be able to cope with a vaginal delivery, the umbilical cord is wrapped around the baby's neck which could cut off its oxygen supply while being born, the cord has prolapsed (slipped) through the cervix and could be closed off by the pressure of the birth canal, the placenta has torn (abrupted), or the baby isn't moving down the birth canal.

Caesarean section is usually done with an epidural, so you will be conscious throughout and will be able to see your baby immediately, and your partner can be with you in the operating theatre. You can ask your doctor to tell you what's going on throughout, and you can listen to music too, but take your own or you may find yourself subjected to your obstetrician's sense of humour (such as a Saw Doctors compilation featuring It Won't Be Tonight, 25 Pounds, and All Over Now).

A small horizontal incision, called a bikini cut, is made above your pubic bone, and a second incision through this into your uterus. The baby is lifted out and quickly checked before being held up for you to see. If the baby is healthy, your partner can hold him while you're repaired – which usually takes around half an hour.

## Avoiding a Caesarean

Even though it's quick and safe, Caesarean birth is not something you'd do for fun, and is usually performed to safeguard either you or your baby. So can you minimize the chances of having one? If you stay fit and healthy obviously that will help. Fewer women with midwifery-led care need Caesareans, so check out your area to see if this is available. This also applies to having a trained doula, or birth companion, attending you. Standing, walking or even sitting can significantly reduce the time you're in labour. Let gravity help. Globally, most women sit or squat to give birth; the only reason we in the west make women lie down is because it's easier for medical staff to see what's going on. And finally, keep up your fluid intake and maybe even eat little and often to maintain your energy levels ("I'll have the pan fried black pudding and cauliflower cream, the beef Wellington on a celeriac mash with a red wine reduction, and then the chocolate mousse with black cherry jus. Oh, and a bottle of the 2001 Waggawagga shiraz").

## Vaginal birth after Caesarean (VBAC)

It used to be thought that once you'd experienced the delights of a Caesarean section, all your subsequent births would be by the same route. But no longer. These days around 70% of mothers have a normal vaginal birth after a Caesarean. That's because, as well as greatly improved surgical techniques, most Caesareans are prompted by a one-off problem which doesn't occur in the next pregnancy. The main concern with a VBAC is that the scar from the Caesarean may open up during the birth and rupture, and in fact this can occur during the pregnancy without causing any problems. Because modern Caesarean sections use a horizontal cut rather than a vertical one, this risk is much reduced and affects less than 1% of women who try VBAC.

## Useful websites/references

http://www.babycentre.co.uk
http://www.marchofdimes.com
http://www.rcog.org.uk
http://www.patient.co.uk
UK patient health information

# 19 Episiotomy

Ah, the unkindest cut of all. Is it really necessary? Once routinely performed by authoritarian doctors, this is now mostly a matter of choice. A cut is made in the perineum, a muscular area between the lower end of the vagina and the anus. You do get a local anaesthetic and most women say they didn't feel it being done. An episiotomy is sometimes required to make the vaginal opening larger, for example if the baby is becoming distressed and needs to be born quickly, or for a forceps or ventouse delivery.

There's no evidence that an episiotomy heals better or more quickly than a spontaneous tear however, and it can in some cases lead to problems with pain, poor healing and incontinence. Midwives much prefer to avoid doing them unless absolutely necessary. Tears are no more painful to heal and may even be less so, and whether you have a tear, an episiotomy, or neither, studies show that your pelvic floor muscles will be equally strong (or weak) 3 months after birth.

A second degree tear or similar sized episiotomy generally takes 2-3 weeks to heal; some authorities say that a natural tear heals more quickly, but it depends on how severe the damage is. Stitches dissolve in around 10 days, but you may feel pain beyond this.

## Useful websites/references

http://www.babycentre.co.uk
http://www.marchofdimes.com
http://www.rcog.org.uk

# 20 Epidurals and other pain relief

An epidural is an injection using a curved needle which is inserted between the vertebrae of your back. A fine tube is passed through the needle which is then removed. You'll need to keep very still while this is being done. A local anaesthetic is injected through the tube and this numbs your lower abdomen. Usually your feet and legs become numb too, and you can't feel your contractions. A small pump is attached to the tube, and either you can control the pain relief yourself, or the pump feeds you regular doses at timed intervals. Over 90% of women get total relief from an epidural, and your mind remains clear, allowing you to maintain awareness and a sense of control. Another advantage is that it can help lower high blood pressure.

Disadvantages include only being anaesthetised down one side, or part of your abdomen remaining sensitive. You'll most likely have a drip in your arm so you can't move about. You may also feel shivery, and you'll probably have a catheter inserted because the numbness means you won't feel the need to go to the toilet.

Labour can be protracted, you may feel you've been "medicalised", there's a higher likelihood of the baby needing a forceps or ventouse delivery, you may have problems urinating after the birth, and if the epidural needle went too far in you'll have a leakage of cerebrospinal fluid which will give you the mother of all headaches.

Up to 15% of women develop a fever after an epidural, and the longer the labour, the higher the risk. Because fever is a sign of infection, your baby is likely to be subjected to blood tests and a spinal tap, given preventive antibiotics and kept in hospital until test results come back. One woman in 5 experiences a drop in blood pressure, requiring corrective drugs. One in 10 babies experiences a serious abnormal heart rate episode due to the epidural.

And you might miss out on all this fun anyway because not all hospitals offer a 24 hour epidural service in England & Wales. Your chances vary from 100% in Oxfordshire, to 58% in the west Midlands, 64% in the south west, to 28% in Wales.

## Pethidine

Pethidine is an analgesic and anti-spasmodic, so it dulls pain and helps you relax. A synthetic version of morphine, it can be given either by injection or intravenously. It's used in the first stage of labour, and is often combined with an anti-emetic, as it can cause nausea. PCA, or patient controlled analgesia, means you can operate the pump delivering pethidine yourself, but not all hospitals offer this. Your midwife can administer it (no need to ask a doctor) and it can be used in a home birth.

Problems with pethidine include making you sleepy (in extreme cases some women miss the party completely and don't even realise they've given birth), you may throw up despite the emetic, some women feel dizzy, labour can be prolonged, and you may feel dozy while contractions are increasing but then suddenly leap into alertness when they peak. As far as your baby is concerned, pethidine can cross the placenta and affect its breathing, and in some cases it can cause convulsions. The baby may need an injection of narcan (naloxone) as soon as it's born to reverse the effects. The baby might be sleepy for the first few days and awkward to feed, and breastfeeding can be more difficult. There is also a possibility that if you have pethidine during labour, your baby may be more likely to develop addictions in later life.

## Meptid

This is not a controlled (addictive) drug, but is a straightforward pain killer or analgesic. The standard dose is 100mg. You can have it any time during the first stage of labour and it is less likely than pethidine to affect your baby's breathing. However, it may make you feel sick or dizzy, and not every hospital uses it.

## Syntometrine

At the 3rd stage of labour you are routinely offered an intramuscular injection of syntometrine (aka syntometrin), which is a blend of oxytocin and ergometrine. This is intended to speed up the delivery of the placenta and prevent post-partum bleeding. PPH, or post-partum haemorrhage, affects 1 in 100,000 women in the UK, which is a very low risk. There is evidence that managed 3rd stage (having the injection, early cutting of the cord, midwife pulling the placenta out) reduces the chances of a mother haemorrhaging by as much as 60%. Because managed 3rd stage speeds things up so much, it can happen that the placenta doesn't have time to detach, so when the midwife pulls on the cord it can snap. If your cervix then closes, the placenta is trapped inside. This can necessitate an epidural or general anaesthetic to remove it. The alternative is physiological 3rd stage, where nature takes her course – and her time, as this lasts 10-60 minutes rather than the 5-15 minutes if you have syntometrine. Advocates of this method feel that a mother should be able to have this time to get to know her baby, allowing the cord to cease pulsating naturally, so that it can be cut later. This means the baby still has an oxygen supply via the cord until it's ready to breathe alone. The risk of a retained placenta is reduced, especially if you suckle the baby during this time: natural oxytocin is released, causing contractions that expel the afterbirth.

## Useful websites/references

http://www.babycentre.co.uk
http://www.aims.org.uk
http://www.birthchoiceuk.com
Good site with maternity statistics etc

http://www.babyworld.co.uk
This site is very useful for regional and local health authority stats.

**http://www.nctpregnancyandbabycare.com/home.asp**
National Childcare Trust

**http://www.babyandkids.co.uk**
**www.nice.org.uk**
Pdf leaflet: Routine antenatal care for healthy pregnant women
Understanding NICE guidance – info for pregnant women, their families and the
public. ISBN: 1-84257-402-7
Published by the National Institute for Clinical Excellence October 2003

**http://www.dh.gov.uk**
Dept of Health site. The Pregnancy Book March 2005 edition
Pdf or browsable, hardcopy. Dept of Health, 31/3/2005. 266528. 152p.

**http://www.marchofdimes.com**
**http://www.rcog.org.uk**

# Part 3
# Newborns

## 21 Heel prick test

This involves taking a blood sample from the heel of the infant to test for cystic fibrosis (CF), phenylketonuria (PKU), and congenital hypothyroidism (CHT). Annually around 1 in 2,500 babies are diagnosed with CF. For both PKU and CHT the number is 250 out of all babies screened per year (around 600,000). You do not have to have this test done if you don't want to.

Phenylketonuria (PKU) is a genetic disorder the incidence of which varies widely, from around 1 in 4,500 in the Irish to fewer than 1 in 100,000 Finns. PKU is typified by the lack of an enzyme called phenylalanine hydroxylase. This leads to a build-up of the amino acid phenylalanine, which has a toxic effect on the central nervous system and can cause brain damage resulting in mental retardation. Treatment involves strict dietary discipline in avoiding foods containing phenylalanine, mostly proteins and starches.

Hypothyroidism is relatively rare – occurring in around 1 in 4,000 babies – and is due to a lack of thyroid hormone. This may be congenital hypothyroidism (CH), usually accounting for 90% of infant cases, in which the thyroid gland is underdeveloped or dysfunctional. In approx 10% of babies the culprit is transient hypothyroidism (TH), where the mother has been treated for thyroid problems or has been exposed to substances which contain iodine. With TH the condition will correct itself. CH leads to inhibited mental development and restricted growth, and treatment involves thyroid hormone replacement, usually in pill form.

The test is done in the first week after birth by piercing the baby's heel with a sharp lancet, then letting the foot hang down to drip blood onto a blood spot card. If you think this sounds painful for the baby, you're darned right. It won't be much fun for you either.

In the UK all babies are screened for PKU and CHT. In some areas babies are also screened for cystic fibrosis, sickle cell disorders and some other conditions.

Screening all new babies for CF is being phased in, to cover all areas of England by April 2007.

It's possible to screen for cystic fibrosis during pregnancy, but this isn't done in the UK. Blood is tested for higher than normal levels of immunoreactive trypsin (IRT), which indicate the presence of CF. It cannot identify whether the baby is just a carrier. The heel prick test is a screening, not a diagnostic test. This means that unusual results do not necessarily indicate your baby has a problem. If the baby has not had a bowel movement in the first 24-48 hours after birth (meconium ileus) this can be a sign that it may have CF.

The heel prick test with regard to cystic fibrosis is a presumptive test: it has a significant rate of false positives, so further confirmatory tests need to be done if it comes up positive.

## Carriers

We all inherit 2 copies of each of our genes: one from mum and one from dad. If 1 or both copies of a gene have a mutation, the function of that gene is altered. If there is only 1 mutated gene in a pair, you're a carrier. This means you won't have the disease yourself, but you are capable of passing it on to your offspring. If your partner also is a carrier, then your baby may inherit 2 mutated genes and can therefore suffer from that particular disease, e.g. cystic fibrosis, phenylketonuria and sickle cell disorders. Being a carrier is quite common: in the UK about 1 in 25 people is a CF carrier.

## The test

It's done by the midwife, and should involve an automated spring loaded lancet because this is quicker and less distressing for the baby. There has been a surprising amount of debate over whether this test really hurts babies or not. Some health professionals claim it doesn't, because newborn babies aren't capable of feeling pain to the same degree as the rest of us. It is noticeable that none of these people has ever stuck a heel prick lancet into themselves to see if it hurts.

## Neonatal pain

An exhaustive examination of neonatal (newborn) pain literature done at the Royal Prince Albert Hospital in New South Wales, Australia, resulted in their Neonatal Pain Policy created in March 2004. The introduction states:

"Neonates, both term and preterm, experience pain and have the right to receive effective and safe pain relief. Compared with the adult, the neonate at birth, whether term or preterm, displays a *hypersensitivity* to sensory stimuli. While self-report ... is regarded as the most reliable estimate of pain and considered the gold standard, neonates cannot verbalise their pain and thus depend on others to recognise, assess and manage their pain."

The italics are mine. I emphasise this because, far from having less sensitivity to pain than an adult, newborn babies are actually more sensitive than us, just less capable of expressing it. Further:

"Common misconceptions concerning newborn pain still exist and include first, the false premise that newborns do not have the neurological substrate for the perception of pain because of lack of myelination, incomplete pain pathways from the periphery to the cortex, or immaturity of the cerebral cortex; second, that newborns do not remember pain, or if they do, it has no adverse effects; third, that it is too dangerous to administer anaesthesia or postoperative analgesia to newborn infants."

The policy goes on to say that pain in neonates is often unrecognised and therefore under treated, and recommends 4 accepted assessment tools for the evaluation of neonate pain: Premature Infant Pain Profile; Neonatal Facial Coding Scale; Neonatal Infant Pain Scale; and the CRIES score: Crying Requires Increased oxygen administration, Increased vital signs, Expression, Sleeplessness.

Sedation is not recommended because it does not decrease pain, and may mask the baby's responses to it. A lack of behavioural responses, such as crying or movement, does not necessarily mean no pain is being felt.

Venepuncture is recommended over heel prick – this is where blood is taken from a vein, usually in the back of the hand. It is less painful for the baby, more efficient, and leads to fewer repeat samples needing to be taken. Because venepuncture requires a skilled and experienced practitioner it may not be practicable for it to be used routinely for testing, but if your baby needs several blood tests you may wish to ask if venepuncture can be used instead of heel prick (1).

A study reported in the Australian Journal of Advanced Nursing compared heel prick to venepuncture with regard to pain. The time taken to collect the sample, and the amount of distress caused to the baby was recorded. 36 babies were involved, and venepuncture was found to be superior in terms of speed and reduced pain for the infant. This is a small study but is supported by research elsewhere (2).

## Lancets

There are 2 methods for doing a heel prick test: a manual lancet, where the nurse pierces the baby's foot; and an automated lancet, which is spring loaded and makes the incision automatically. Research has shown that the automated lancet is by far the best method to use: it is quicker, causes less pain, and reduces the need for repeat puncturing. As an example, an experiment done in Finland in 2000 tested both methods on 100 preterm infants in a randomised blind study.

To obtain the required amount of blood, the conventional lancet needed on average 2.6 times more punctures. It caused more bruising of the heel (100% v 84%), more inflammation (79% v 53%), and more bruising of the leg and ankle (92% v 53%). There was no difference in how quickly skin healed. Researchers concluded that the automated lancet was less traumatic for collecting repeated samples from preterm infants. **(3)**

## What works?

So if you take the advice to have the heel prick test, there you are holding your baby who is about to experience some significant pain. What can you do? Topical analgesics like anaesthetic creams and gels don't help – in fact they can make things worse because they restrict blood vessels, reducing the blood flow.

The Neonatal Pain Policy, backed by several pieces of research, states that giving your baby a 12 – 24% sucrose solution 2 minutes before the procedure has the best analgesic result. You can also provide sensory distraction while the test is being done. This means cuddling the baby, stroking and soothing it, feeding it, and taking its attention away from the pain in its foot. Heel warming is largely ineffective and only prolongs the experience, and squeezing the heel to increase or encourage blood flow increases the pain significantly and should not be necessary.

## Premature babies

For preterm babies who may need lots of heel prick tests, the heel can become very tender and sore because only a limited area of the foot is considered safe to use. Recent research has suggested that this is not the case, and the whole area of the sole of the foot can safely be used **(4)**.

# References

**1** RPA Newborn Care Protocol Book
Royal Prince Alfred Hospital (New South Wales, Australia)

Neonatal Pain Policy Created: March 2004
Main author: Heather Jeffery

**2** Australian Journal of Advanced Nursing 1999 Sept-Nov;17(1):30-6
Venepuncture versus heel prick for the collection of the Newborn Screening Test.
Logan PW.
Clinical Management Centre, Warrnambool and District Base Hospital, Victoria, Australia.

**3** Archives of Disease in Childhood: Fetal & Neonatal Edition 2001;84:F53-F55 ( January )

An automatic incision device for obtaining blood samples from the heels of preterm infants causes less damage than a conventional manual lancet

H Vertanen a, V Fellman b, M Brommels c, L Viinikka a

a Department of Clinical Chemistry, Helsinki University Central Hospital, Helsinki, Finland, b Hospital for Children and Adolescents, Helsinki University Central Hospital, c Department of Public Health, University of Helsinki, Helsinki

**4** Archives of Disease in Childhood, Neonatal Edition 1999;80:F243-F245 (May)

Ultrasound study of heel to calcaneum depth in neonates

Anoo Jain,a Nicholas Rutter b

a Department of Neonatal Medicine, Nottingham City Hospital, Nottingham NG5 1PB, b Division of Child Health, School of Human Development, Queen's Medical Centre, Nottingham

# 22  Vitamin K

This is a blood clotting agent. Vitamin K deficiency bleeding (VKDB) affects around 1 in 10,000 newborn babies, which means they can have nose or mouth bleeds, or internal bleeding, especially inside the head, which can have serious and even fatal consequences. However, this is a very low-risk, and some people have questioned whether it warrants all babies routinely being given vitamin K supplements. You have a choice as to whether or not you accept this treatment for your baby.

VKDB is classified into early, classical, and late, depending on when it occurs. Early VKDB is usually associated with antenatal drugs that interfere with vitamin K metabolism. Classical and late VKDB are connected to breastfeeding and malabsorption (the baby not absorbing enough vitamin K via feeding).

The Department of Health recommends that breastfed babies are given either 1 injection of vitamin K soon after birth, or oral vitamin K twice within the 1st week, followed by another oral dose at 1 month. For bottle fed babies it's either the injection or 2 oral doses in the 1st week.

Why more for breastfed babies? Some research was done that found low levels of vitamin K in breast milk, but this has been challenged on the grounds that when the study was done, it was at a time when women were encouraged to limit feeding in the first few days. This led to babies not getting much of the hind milk, which is fattier and has the highest concentrations of vitamin K (along with colostrum). Thus the research may be based on erroneous information.

Also, the levels of vitamin K were compared to those in cow's milk, but there's no reason to assume that cow's milk and human breast milk should be comparable in this way. If babies have low levels of vitamin K compared to adults, this is to be expected – they're smaller. It's possible that babies' levels are perfectly normal.

## What's the best way to deliver vitamin K?

If you do go with having the supplementation, what's best? Various studies have been done, and the consensus seems to be that the intramuscular injection is more effective, especially in the prevention of late VKDB. Otherwise, 3 oral doses are necessary.

A 6 year surveillance study done in Switzerland looked at whether 2 or 3 oral doses of vitamin K were more effective. An oral dose of 2mg was given on the 1st and 4th day after birth. Of 475,000 births, there were no cases of early (<24 hrs), 1 case of classical (2-7 days), and 18 cases of late (1-12 weeks) VKDB. In 13 of the 18 late cases, there was pre-existing liver disease. In 4 of the 18, the parents had refused vitamin K treatment. In the remaining 1 case, the baby had received treatment and did not have liver disease. The study concluded that 2 oral doses is not enough for prevention, and Swiss protocol has been changed to include a 3rd dose given at 4 weeks of age. (1)

## Contraindications

A preservative, benzyl alcohol, is often included in commercial preparations of vitamin K, or in the diluent (stuff used to mix it with). This can cause an allergic reaction in new infants so it's important to ensure that the form used for babies is preservative free. Contraindications for adult use of vitamin K injections include rare but possibly fatal allergic reaction, and state that the injectable form of the vitamin should only be used when the oral form is not available. It also says that intramuscular injection can have "very serious" side effects. None of these are mentioned in the research done on babies.

# Useful websites/references

www.medicinenet.com
http://www.babycentre.co.uk
http://www.marchofdimes.com

# Other references

1   European Journal of Pediatrics

Prevention of vitamin K deficiency bleeding with oral mixed micellar phylloqui-
none: results of a 6-year surveillance in Switzerland.
Schubiger G, Berger TM, Weber R, Banziger O, Laubscher B; Swiss Paediatric
Surveillance Unit.
Department of Paediatrics, Children's Hospital of Lucerne, Switzerland

# Part 4

# Babies

## 23  Car safety

First, mum: by law, all pregnant women must wear a seat belt when travelling in a car, whether driving, or sitting front or back. Put the diagonal strap between your breasts, over the breastbone, with the strap going over your shoulder, not resting on your neck. The lap belt should be flat on the thighs, under your bump and over your pelvis. Wear the belt as tight as you can bear it. Lap-only belts should be avoided, as they can cause serious injuries to the baby if there is sudden deceleration.

### Scary bits

In 2004 the number of 0–4 year old children killed as passengers in cars was 15. One hundred and twenty three were seriously injured and 2,077 were slightly injured. The total of children 0-11 killed or injured was 7,696. These figures are not as high as one might expect, but as with any statistics, the numbers don't matter when the 1 in 10,000,000 is yours.

Nearly all road accidents involve human error, usually on the part of the driver. The main reason why men have car accidents is impatience. The main reason why women do is that they get distracted. Unsurprisingly perhaps, the morning and afternoon school runs are peak times for accidents involving children.

## Car seats

Around 70% of child car seats are incorrectly fitted, mainly because of poor instructions, or because the seat is not compatible with the model of car. Bearing this in mind, the first thing to do is to find out which seats work with your car. If you are buying from new, the shop should be able to advise you on this, and some will let you try the seat in your car before you buy it.

RoSPA (Royal Society for the Prevention of Accidents) recommends that your baby should be placed in a rearward facing seat or infant carrier rather than a front facing one. This is the safest way for it to travel and it should not go into a forward facing seat until it weighs at least 9kgs and can sit up unaided.

*Never* put a baby seat in the front seat of your car if it has a passenger airbag fitted. This could be fatal.

In September 2006 new regulations governing the use of child car seats came into force. With regard to children under three, the rules are:

- If carried [i.e. travelling] in the front seat, an appropriate child restraint must be used (the adult seat belt is not sufficient). Children under 3 years old may not travel in the front unless they are in a child restraint.

- If carried in the rear seat, an appropriate child restraint must be used if available.

- If an appropriate restraint is fitted in the front of the car, but not the rear, children under 3 years old must sit in the front and use that restraint. You can move the restraint from the front to the rear if you wish. Rearward facing seats are designed to be used in the rear as well as the front. You should always put a rearward facing baby seat in the rear if a front passenger airbag is fitted.

*(From the RoSPA website)*

# ISOFIX

Not a new type of glue, this is in fact "International Standards Organisation FIX." The idea behind it is to make the fitting of child seats into cars by normal parents, who don't have a degree in engineering, much easier.

It works like this: ISOFIX points are built into the cars while on the assembly line. Child seat manufacturers include ISOFIX fitting points on the seats. This will enable the seat to be plugged into position with the minimum of faffing, effing and fluffing.

ISOFIX isn't finalised yet, but there are some specific car models and child seats available that do include the new system. Britax make a Duo ISOFIX that can be used in over 80 models of car.

## New or second hand?

Baby seats and infant carriers are often rather expensive. Should you consider buying second hand? Official advice is don't, because if the seat has been involved in a crash, its structural integrity may be compromised. There could be cracks in the frame, or other damage not visible to the naked eye. Only if you know the history of the seat, i.e. it belonged to family or friends, should you consider buying it.

You can get in touch with your local council's road safety department to see if they run a child seat discount scheme – some do. They may also have a seat hire facility.

In 2003 the Consumer's Association and the AA Motoring Trust tested 52 child car seats available across Europe. These tests were more rigorous than the standard safety tests, and included impact at 40 mph, and side impact (amazingly, the new ECE Regulation 44.03 doesn't cover side impact testing).

Booster seats were the main problem, and you'll be glad to hear that seats designed for babies and children up to 4 years old came out very well.

## Useful websites/references

**http://www.childcarseats.org.uk/**
Produced by RoSPA with the support of the Department for Transport

**http://www.theaa.com**
AA website

**http://www.britax.co.uk**
Lots of information, car fit-finder

# 24 Sudden Infant Death Syndrome (SIDS)

Sudden Infant Death Syndrome, aka cot death, is not a disease but a diagnosis – it's what's left when there is no explanation for the death of newborn or very young babies. There is no 'cause', and thus no cure. Therefore the approach is preventive: what can you do to minimise the risk for your baby?

Around 350 babies a year in the UK have deaths that are ascribed to SIDS. There may be a possible physical trigger, such as under development of vital regulating systems; or environmental factors like smoking; or the way the baby sleeps. Research is ongoing as to whether genetic or anatomical problems may also contribute to these unexplained deaths.

Most at risk are babies who:
- Are premature
- Are low birthweight
- Are up to 1 year old, especially below 4-6 months
- Have a previous sibling who died of SIDS
- Have a mother who smokes or takes drugs
- Have a mother who was under 20 for her 1st pregnancy
- Live in a smoky environment

Other factors include being put down to sleep on their front or side, overheating, and having had a life threatening episode, especially one connected to breathing problems.

In 1991 the Foundation for the Study of Infant Deaths (FSID) began a campaign called Reduce the Risk to reduce the number of cot deaths, and since then these have decreased by over 70%. SIDS is now linked to lower socio-economic status, reflecting perhaps that those in most need of preventive advice aren't getting it.

## 'Back to sleep'

The most crucial thing you can do to help your baby is to put it down to sleep on its back. There are various reasons behind this: babies who lie on their fronts may over inhale carbon dioxide; they may breathe in toxins from the mattress; they may have an under developed regulatory mechanism for their blood pressure; they may restrict an artery in their neck; they may suffocate in soft bedding. They may also overheat, as the body is more able to lose heat from the front than the back, so the baby can cool down more readily if it's lying on its back.

In a way, none of these matters: we don't know which if any of these things a particular baby might suffer from, so the bottom line is, keep it on its back anyway. It's been proven to help lower the risk.

The Feet to Foot guideline advises that you put your baby to sleep so that its feet are close to the foot of its cot. This helps prevent it from wriggling down under the covers.

Safety recommendations state that to avoid suffocation babies should sleep on firm mattresses, with the bottom sheet and blankets tucked in securely. Also no fluffy things, cot bumpers or soft toys in the cot with the baby. Avoid letting it sleep on beanbags and similar squashy surfaces for the same reason.

Babies can't regulate their body temperature when they're small, and overheating increases the risk of cot death. The ambient temperature in the bedroom should be around 18°C (64°F) and parents are advised not to cover the baby's head when it's in bed.

Another standard guideline is that for the first 6 months of your baby's life you should keep it in the same room as you at night to reduce the chances of it having breathing or other problems that may otherwise go unnoticed.

## Dummies

Sucking a dummy (or pacifier, as they call it across the pond) has been shown to reduce the risk of SIDS, mainly, it seems, because dummies have sticky-out bits that stop the baby from rolling onto its face. The constant sucking action may also strengthen neural pathways in the baby's brain connected to its breathing development. The most significant improvement in decreased risk using dummies has been in circumstances where the baby is exposed to adverse conditions such as tobacco smoke (cigarettes, pipes, cigars, smoke signals, Native American peace pipe ceremonies etc) on a regular basis.

## Other risk factors

A Norwegian study examined 1,483,857 births between 1969-1995 to see if there was a link between SIDS and low socio-economic status. The absolute risk for SIDS among babies whose mothers had low education increased by 0.51 per 1000 births, compared to the risk for babies of highly educated mothers which decreased by 0.56 per 1000. The relative SIDS risk for babies of low education mothers increased from 1.02 in the 1970s to 2.39 in the 80s and 5.63 in the 90s. (1)

A Swedish study reported in Acta Paediatrica March 2006 found that though the practice of putting babies to sleep on their backs, and mothers stopping smoking, has reduced the risks of SIDS, other factors have become more prominent. Side sleeping is a risk, as is bed sharing if the baby is below 2-3 months old (especially if the mother is a smoker), while the use of pacifiers (dummies) is beneficial. Any nicotine use should be avoided during pregnancy and breastfeeding, and "replacement of maternal smoking with nicotine substitutes is not harmless."

I take this last comment to mean that nicotine gum and patches are considered to have some risk attached to them, and have seen this mentioned in other research, but what that risk is has not been made clear. Nicotine in any form is not a good thing, but at least with nicotine replacement there's nothing else harmful added as there is in cigarettes.**(2)**

Another significant factor that increases the risk of SIDS is if a woman has had a SIDS baby before. A Cambridge study examined 258,096 women in Scotland who had consecutive births between 1985-2001, using linked UK databases. This found that women who had had a baby who died from SIDS were more likely in their next pregnancy to have a baby that was either small for gestational age (SGA), or premature. Also that if the previous baby had been SGA or premature, this increased the risk of SIDS for the next child. Small or premature babies were the result of obstetrical complications which were likely to recur in future pregnancies. **(3)**

## Bed sharing

Is it safe for your baby to sleep in your bed (co-sleep) with you? The scientific consensus seems to be that if either parent drinks, does drugs, or takes medication that causes drowsiness, don't ever go to sleep with your baby. Not in bed, not on the sofa, not anywhere. In such circumstances people sleep more heavily, and are more likely to roll onto a baby without realising it. This risk also applies even if you're just very tired, or are a heavy sleeper (what, with a new baby in the house?) or your baby is small/low birthweight or was premature.

However, other schools of thought say that when co-sleeping, a parent can be responsive to the baby's breathing and movement patterns, and there are the obvious emotional bonding advantages. And mothers have been sharing beds with their babies for centuries. A useful tip is for both of you to be naked: skin is touch sensitive and clothing isn't.

The Foundation for the Study of Infant Deaths (FSID) recently funded a study called "Major epidemiological changes in sudden infant death syndrome: a 20 year population based study in the UK." This found that the incidence of co-sleeping associated infant deaths had increased by 40%. Around 135 babies a year die when in a bed with a parent. However, they do make the provisos mentioned above, from which you could draw the conclusion that if you don't take drugs, don't drink, and don't behave irresponsibly, co-sleeping is probably all right, especially if it doesn't mean an all-nighter, but just short term cuddles and feeds.

The study mentioned above looked at data collected between 1984 and 2003. They note that over the past 20 years, the proportion of babies who died while bedsharing with parents increased from 12% to 50%. But the actual number of SIDS deaths from co-sleeping has halved. The reason for the increase may be that there were fewer deaths of babies that slept alone, rather than a rise in babies who shared a bed; also there was an increase in deaths related to babies and parents sleeping together on a sofa. Significantly, the proportion of SIDS deaths in families from deprived socio-economic backgrounds has increased from 47% to 54%, and the number of mothers who smoke during pregnancy has risen from 57% to 86%. The prevalence of preterm babies has risen from 12% to 34%, and first born babies are now the largest at-risk group. Bedsharing is now more likely to involve younger babies, and fewer are breastfed. **(4)**

Infant deaths from sofa sharing are on the increase too: to 30 a year. Again, this is linked to more vulnerable households – for which read: parents/carers who use drugs, drink a lot, and lead chaotic, fragile lifestyles.

FSID recommends that the safest place for a baby to sleep is in a cot beside mum and dad's bed for the first 6 months.

The Ulster Medical Journal reported in Jan 2005 on a study of Northern Ireland autopsy reports between April 1996 and August 2001. This was to evaluate the incidence of SUDI (Sudden Unexpected Death in Infancy) involving bed sharing. 43 cases of SUDI were identified, with a further 2 cases due to suffocation from overlaying. 32 of the 45 were less than 4 months old. 30 of the 45 had been bed sharing: 19 in an adult bed, 11 on a sofa or armchair. SUDI was twice as frequent at weekends, as were co-sleeping deaths, and 49% of SUDI happened in summer. The study says "While sharing a place of sleep per se may not increase risk of death, our findings may be linked to factors such as habitual smoking, consumption of alcohol or illicit drugs..." **(5)**

## Space oddity

Here's an interesting idea: the connection between astronauts and foetuses. Published in Medical Hypotheses 2006 "Sudden infant death syndrome (SIDS): microgravity and inadequate sensory stimulation" postulates that astronauts and foetuses experience very similar environments – at least until the foetus is 26 weeks old. After that, as a baby becomes heavier, its physical systems have to learn to adapt to coping with weight and gravity. If a baby is born prematurely, it misses out on the development caused by gravitational loading, and some of its systems remain immature. The deconditioning experienced by astronauts in antigravity is the reverse of this loading process. A growth retarded foetus, the argument goes, may have been deprived of "the mechanical dimension of uterine wall pressure." I take this to mean that gravity and pressure in utero contribute to the development of the foetus. NASA research which looked into the deconditioning effects of antigravity was based on the insight that the physiological effects of space travel are almost identical to the adjustments the body makes when lying down. It has been found that in some babies who died of SIDS, there may have been problems with the equalisation of blood pressure when the baby lies down. **(6)**

Following on from this, I note a study done in the Dept of Psychiatry, Columbia University College of Physicians and Surgeons, New York. This looked at heart rate responses to head-up tilting in babies (raising them from a flat position to an upright one). 54 babies, including newborns and 2-4 months old, were tested. Their heart rates were measured during slow and rapid tilting. Newborn babies' rates increased at both speeds, whereas 2-4 month old babies didn't. In other words, newborns reacted as adults would, but slightly older babies don't adjust their heart rates (and therefore blood pressure) to being tilted. The conclusion was that "There are significant early developmental changes in cardiac responses to hypotensive challenge." Hypotensive = abnormally low blood pressure. The tilt test may "provide a standardised method for assessing autonomic competence during the period of maximum vulnerability to SIDS". (7) Maybe the astronaut theory isn't so mad after all.

## Useful websites/references

Foundation for the Study of Infant Death (FSID)

**http://sids.org.uk**
FSID runs a Helpline (020 7233 2090) for parents and carers with questions about safe baby care. The Helpline also supports anyone who has experienced the sudden death of a baby.

## Other references

1  The Lancet 2006; 367:314-319
   DOI:10.1016/S0140-6736(06)67968-3
   Major epidemiological changes in sudden infant death syndrome: a 20-year population-based study in the UK
   Peter S Blair, Peter Sidebotham, P Jeremy Berry, Margaret Evans and Peter J Fleming

2  Acta Paediatrica 2006 Mar;95(3):260-2
   Stop SIDS—sleeping solitary supine, sucking soother, stopping smoking substitutes.
   Alm B, Lagercrantz H, Wennergren G.
   Department of Paediatrics, Goteborg University, Queen Silvia Children's Hospital, Goteborg, Sweden.

3  Lancet 2005 Dec 17;366(9503):2107-11
   Sudden infant death syndrome and complications in other pregnancies.
   Smith GC, Wood AM, Pell JP, Dobbie R.
   Department of Obstetrics and Gynaecology, Cambridge University, Rosie Hospital, Cambridge UK

4  International Journal of Epidemiology 2006 Mar 23; Epub ahead of print
   Post-neonatal mortality in Norway 1969-95: a cause-specific analysis.
   Arntzen A, Samuelsen SO, Daltveit AK, Stoltenberg C.
   Faculty of Social Science, Vestfold University College, PO Box 2243, N-3103 Tonsberg, Norway.

**5** Ulster Medical Journal 2005 Jan;75(1):65-71
Sudden unexpected death in infancy: place and time of death.
Glasgow JF, Thompson AJ, Ingram PJ.
Royal Belfast Hospital for Sick Children

**6** Medical hypotheses 2006;66(5):920-4 Epub 2005 Dec 27
Sudden infant death syndrome (SIDS): Microgravity and inadequate sensory stimulation.
Reid GM.
Gilchrist Street, Te Aroha, New Zealand

**7** Acta Paediatrica 2006 Jan;95(1):77-81
Developmental changes in infant heart rate responses to head-up tilting.
Myers MM, Gomez-Gribben E, Smith KS, Tseng A, Fifer WP.
Department of Psychiatry, Columbia University College of Physicians and Surgeons, New York, USA

# 25 MMR vaccination

Scaremongery or scientific fact – is there a link between the MMR jab and autism? Well, I can only give you the evidence I've seen, and then you must make up your own mind. I feel it's important to reiterate that at this point, because this is a particularly inflammatory subject. Autistic spectrum disorder (ASD) is the term used for a range of autism problems, including Asperger's syndrome.

## The case for the prosecution

Dr Andrew Wakefield and colleagues reported on research they had done into a possible connection between autistic regression, intestinal problems and the MMR vaccine in the Lancet of February 1998. Twelve children were involved in the study, 6 of whom had manifested autistic symptoms within 2 weeks of being vaccinated with the MMR jab. The study states "We did not prove an association between measles, mumps, and rubella vaccine and the syndrome described." The interpretation of the research said "We identified associated gastrointestinal disease and developmental regression in a group of previously normal children, which was generally associated in time with possible environmental triggers."
(1)

Since then, controversy has raged. In February 2004 the Lancet reported on an apparent conflict of interest: Dr Wakefield had received £55,000 from attorneys via the Legal Aid Board to support claims made by parents regarding the MMR autism connection. In March 2004 the Lancet published a retraction by 10 of the 13 authors of the original report. The retraction stated "We wish to make it clear that in this paper no causal link was established between MMR vaccine and autism as the data were insufficient," but the retraction was partial, maintaining that the idea of there being a possible link between intestinal illness and autism is a serious one, worthy of further investigation.

The MMR vaccine can cause febrile seizures, probably associated with vaccine induced fever. In a Danish study involving all children born 1991-1998 (540,000), 440,000 (82%) had the MMR vaccine. 17,986 children had at least 1 febrile seizure, of which 973 occurred within 2 weeks. The rate of 1st seizure was 10% higher in vaccinated children, and seizures happened more frequently in the 1st and 2nd weeks after vaccination. For vaccinated children with a history of febrile seizures, the additional risk within the first 2 weeks increased from 12 in 1000 to 31 in 1000.

Febrile seizures are convulsions brought on by fever in babies and small children. About 1 in 25 children will have at least one seizure. The majority are harmless, and most children grow out of them.

A study done at Tokyo Medical University in 2000 examined whether the measles virus could be found in the gut of patients with Crohn's disease and children who had developed autism post-vaccination with MMR. The researchers wanted to know if this was the result of wild (ie ordinary) measles, or the vaccine strain. Eight Crohn's disease patients, 3 ulcerative colitis patients, and 9 children with autistic enterocolitis were included, plus 8 healthy controls. One CD patient, 1 UC patient, and 3 autism children were found positive for the presence of measles virus. Controls were all negative. The CD patient showed positive for the wild variant of measles. The UC and autism children showed positive for the vaccine strain. **(2)**

Another study done at Utah State University 2002 suggested that autistic children experienced an "inappropriate antibody response" to MMR, and particularly to the measles component of it, which "might be related to pathogenesis of autism" (pathogenesis = the start of a disease). Scientists used serum samples from 125 autistic children and 92 controls. Analysis showed the presence of an unusual MMR antibody in 75 (60%) of the autistic children but not in the controls. Also, over 90% of the MMR antibody-positive samples in the autistic children also showed positive for myelin basic protein (MBP) autoantibodies. MBP is an "ingredient" of the central nervous system. Again, the controls were negative. The study concludes that there is a strong association between MMR and central nervous system autoimmunity in autism (autoimmunity = the immune system turns on the body's own cells as if they were germs). **(3)**

## Thiomersal (aka Thimerosal)

This is a fungicide and preservative often sprayed on grain and sometimes used in vaccines, and is an organic compound containing 49.6% ethylmercury. Concerned parents who believe there is a connection between autism and MMR have cited this preservative as a possible trigger.

Thiomersal (or the US version, thimerosal) breaks down into 2 components in the body: sodium thiosalicylate and ethylmercury. It is eventually metabolised into inorganic mercury. Mercury crosses the blood-brain barrier (and the placenta) and is distributed mainly in the central nervous system, liver, kidneys and skin.

I quote from the University of Illinois at Chicago (UIC) College of Pharmacy drug information center: "There currently are no guidelines that set acceptable exposure levels to ethylmercury, the main mercurial component of thimerosal. The data used to determine toxicity potential have been correlated with levels of methylmercury, *not* ethylmercury. Since there is a lack of comparative data on metabolism, elimination, toxicity, and risk to fetus between ethylmercury and methylmercury, there are still questions as to whether or not exposure to ethylmercury poses the same threat as exposure to methylmercury."

## A change in policy

In June 1999, the Agency for the Evaluation of Medicinal Products (EMEA), a European body, completed an 18-month inquiry into the risks and benefits of using thimerosal in vaccines. EMEA concluded that "although there is no evidence of harm caused by the level of exposure from vaccines, it would be prudent to promote the general use of vaccines without thimerosal."

The FDA's Center for Biologics Evaluation & Research (CBER) found that thimerosal was present in over 30 licensed vaccines in the US in concentrations of 0.003% to 0.01%. According to the agency's calculations, an infant six months old who got all vaccine doses on schedule would receive a total of 187.5 micrograms of mercury. This exceeded the limit set by the EPA (Environmental Protection Agency).

Although the FDA review found no evidence of harm caused by the amount of thimerosal in vaccinations beyond minor local skin reactions, the American Academy of Pediatrics (AAP), the American Academy of Family Physicians (AAFP), the Advisory Committee on Immunization Practices (ACIP), and the United States Public Health Service (PHS) issued a joint statement regarding thimerosal content of vaccines in 1999, establishing a goal of removing thimerosal from all infant vaccines as soon as possible.

Thiomersal is now no longer used in the preparation of any vaccines given in the UK.

## The case for the defence

I've used a comprehensive report by the excellent medical science site Bandolier for a lot of this, because they've done a better job of collating, critiquing and comparing than I ever could.

The risk factors for autism aren't well understood. There's some evidence, for example, that it occurs more often in the families of scientists or professionals. There's also an indication that it may be associated with maternal smoking in early pregnancy, or Caesarean birth, or being born outside the fortunate realms of Europe and North America. The implications are that intrauterine and neonatal factors are important contributing elements. Some researchers think there is a connection to infectious agents, others that there is a genetic component. It seems there may be no single cause of autism, either genetic or environmental.

Autism is on the increase in many countries. An example from London looked at 567 children diagnosed with autistic spectrum disorder (ASD) born 1979-1998. Using children aged 5-14, at the end of 2000 the prevalence of ASD was 19 per 10,000. There was some evidence of a reduction in age of diagnosis over time. Provisional diagnosis was made at 3.5 years in 1985 but 3.0 years by 1995 for childhood and atypical autism (unusual symptoms or features). For Asperger's syndrome, provisional diagnosis was made at 6.0 years in 1985 but at 4.9 years by 1995.

In 44 of 106 children with childhood or atypical autism a specific trigger was mentioned as a possible cause. These were:

- 13: household or social change (like birth of a sibling)
- 12: vaccination (MMR in 8 of the 12)
- 7: viral or bacterial infection
- 7: seizures
- 2: after surgery
- 3: other causes

After excluding unvaccinated cases and those vaccinated when aged over 24 months, MMR was mentioned as a trigger in 6 out of 30 (20%) after August 1997 when the MMR theory of a link with autism was first publicised, and in 2 out of 46 (4%) previous to that date. The trend in diagnosis flattened after about 1991 at about 2.6 per 1000 live births for childhood and atypical autism. There was a levelling off in the number of autism cases during the early 1990s. Neither this, nor the previous increase was related to any change in the rate of MMR vaccination. Bandolier states "...it is worthwhile noting the features, at least in the popular and media mind, that associated MMR with autism. They included the belief that:

- Autism rates had increased owing to introduction of MMR.
- MMR vaccination led to regression; meaning that children who

were developing normally regressed in their development after MMR vaccination.

- MMR vaccination caused a form of autism associated with bowel disorders.
- MMR, but not single vaccines, overwhelmed the immune system.

A huge amount of research of high quality and validity has been assembled subsequently, none of which supports any of these contentions."

I don't want to deluge you with a load of scientific studies, so will use just a few to illustrate the scientific consensus that the MMR jab is safe.

## The Finnish study

In Finland, before immunisation, it was observed that up to a quarter of soldiers in the army had clinical mumps. This was a significant cause of infertility in the general population, and mumps was a major cause of hearing impairment and later deafness in children.

About 1 in 1000 people a year had rubella, which also causes impaired hearing in children, and congenital rubella syndrome in the unborn foetus. This results in miscarriage, stillbirth and severe birth defects, while of those born alive, up to 20% have CRS. The resulting congenital defects include cataracts, heart disease, deafness and mental retardation.

In 1982 a determined effort was put into a vaccination programme, using a triple MMR vaccine. Coverage was over 95%. The number of cases of measles was at 5000 to 15,000 before the vaccination programme was implemented. Since 1985 the number of cases has dropped dramatically, and in 1996 they reached zero. For mumps and rubella the pre-vaccination cases numbered a few thousands to a few tens of thousands per year, but fell, post-vaccination, to a few hundreds or tens. Since 1997 the only recorded cases have been brought in from outside the country.

To examine possible harm resulting from vaccination, the Finnish National Board of Health started a long-term country-wide surveillance system to detect serious adverse events associated with MMR.

From a population of 1.8 million people having 3 million vaccinations, the total number of reported vaccine associated events was 437. Of these, potentially serious events numbered 169, of whom 79 went to hospital. These 169 cases were thoroughly examined. About half of them could be put down to other factors, such as other vaccinations given with the MMR. No event had an incidence of more than 1 case per 100,000 doses of vaccine. There were no cases of autism, Crohn's disease, ulcerative colitis or any chronic disorder affecting the gastrointestinal tract.

## The Japanese study

In 1989 the MMR vaccine was introduced in Japan, but 4 years later it was terminated due to problems with production, and only single vaccines were used subsequently. This in effect is a real life test of whether autism diagnoses fell after the cessation of MMR usage, as would be expected if there were a link. The study was conducted in Yokohama on 300,000 people. Children had routine check-ups at 4, 18 and 36 months. At 18 months about 90% of children took part in the programme, and those who were missed could be referred by nurseries, paediatric clinics and other services. The programme began in 1987, 2 years before the introduction of the MMR vaccine.

Over the whole period, and with full follow-up to age 7 in children born 1988-1996, 278 children developed ASD (autistic spectrum disorder), 158 autism, and 120 other autism disorders – a total of 556. 70% of children born in 1988 received the MMR vaccine, falling over the years to 1.8% in 1992. The incidence of all ASDs, and of autism, continued to rise after the MMR vaccine was discontinued. The incidence of autism was higher in children born after 1992 who were not vaccinated, than in children born before

1992 who were. The levels of autism associated with regression remained the same during and post MMR use.

## New variant MMR-induced autism

It has been suggested that the MMR vaccine causes a new type of autism. This is a combination of developmental regression (where a healthy child starts to lose previously acquired abilities such as talking) and gastrointestinal symptoms manifesting soon after immunisation. The main claims are that there is a new phenotype (outward physical manifestation) of autism involving these 2 factors, that this is responsible for increases in autism rates, and that it is associated with biological findings that suggest persistent measles infection.

These claims have been tested by a UK study using information on three sets of children. Group 1 had 97 children with pervasive developmental disorders (PDD) from Staffordshire born between 1992 and 1995. These included 26 with autistic disorder, atypical autism in 56, and Asperger's syndrome in 13. All had been vaccinated with MMR.

Two clinical samples for comparison were from the Maudsley Hospital. Group 2 included 99 patients with a diagnosis of autism, born 1954-1979, so not exposed to MMR. Group 3 had 68 children born 1987-1996 with a confirmed diagnosis of PDD, and exposed to MMR. There was no difference in the mean age of first parental concern (ie when symptoms were noticed) in the three study samples, which was about 19 months.

In two samples for which information on regressive autism was available, there was no difference in the proportion of children with any form of regressive autism whether exposed to MMR or not. Parents with children with regression did not become concerned at an earlier age than parents of children without regression.

There was no association between regression and gastrointestinal symptoms. Such symptoms were reported for 19 children, with constipation being the most common, followed by abdominal pain, bloody stools, and diarrhoea. Bloody stools were mostly temporary and associated with constipation. No child had inflammatory bowel disorder, or medical investigations for bowel syndromes. No association was found between gastrointestinal symptoms and regression. Only two children in the whole sample (2%) had both gastrointestinal symptoms and regression, lower than what could be expected by chance.

The authors of this study go on to point out that regression in autism is not new. In a review of the literature they demonstrate regression rates of 22% to 50% in studies between 1963 and 1998. The variation between studies is what might be expected by chance given the small numbers of some of the studies, but it is clear that regression occurred in children with autism long before MMR. In this study regression occurred in 18% of autistic children in a pre-MMR sample and in 16% of autistic children in a post-MMR sample. There is no evidence for any increase in regression, any association between gastrointestinal symptoms and regression, nor any change in the descriptions of autism before or after the MMR vaccination was introduced.

No country in the world recommends giving the 3 vaccines separately. 33 European countries, plus Canada, Australia, New Zealand and the USA, all use the MMR vaccine.

## The Danish study

From 1970 the only vaccine being used in Denmark containing thiomersal was a whole-cell pertussis (whooping cough) vaccine. This was used until March 1992 when the vaccine was reformulated without thiomersal and used until January 1997. Inoculations were given at 5 and 9 weeks, and 10 months, and had the equivalent of 25 micrograms of ethylmercury in the 1st dose, and 50 micrograms in the other doses. Of a cohort (group) of 467,450 children, there were 440 cases of autism (average age at diagnosis 4.7 years) and 878 cases of ASD (average age at diagnosis 6 years).

95.6% of children were vaccinated at least once, 89% twice, and 63% received all 3 doses. There was no association between use of thiomersal and the risk of developing autism or ASD. Nor was there any dose-response with increasing exposure over 3 doses.

A recent piece of research (2005) at Duke University Medical Center has discovered the first evidence that complex genetic interactions account for autism risk. This involves GABA receptor genes, which are involved in "off switches" for nerves in the brain. GABA is a neurotransmitter that inhibits neurological response, telling the body to slow down. So the GABA system is a sort of information filter that prevents the body from becoming over stimulated. One of the GABA receptor genes, GABRA4, participates in the origin of autism. It seems to increase autism risk by interacting with a second gene, GABRB1. It's early days, but this could be significant for future treatment of autism. **(4)**

Here's an extract from a letter sent in October 2001 to health professionals from the Chief Medical Officer, Chief Nursing Officer and Chief Pharmaceutical Officer:

2.1 An issue which has gained recent media attention is that of thiomersal in vaccines and possible links to neurodevelopmental disorders, including autism.

2.2 Thiomersal is a mercury based preservative used in some vaccines to prevent microbial contamination or as an inactivating agent to produce killed vaccines. It has been used in vaccines for over 60 years. It has played an important role in maintaining the safety of vaccines.

2.3 The only vaccines used in the routine UK childhood immunisation programme which have contained thiomersal as an excipient in the final product are DTP and DT vaccines...*There is no, and never has been any, thiomersal in any MMR, Hib, oral polio, meningitis C conjugate or BCG vaccines used in the UK.* [my italics]

2.4 There is no doubt that methyl mercury in high doses is

neurotoxic. However, the levels of exposure to thiomersal (which contains ethyl mercury) in vaccines in the UK do not constitute 'high doses'. The amounts of thiomersal in the UK schedule are lower than those in the United States, where the routine programme has recently involved many more vaccines which did contain thiomersal. By 6 months of age, the US schedule provided children with more than twice the amount of thiomersal experienced in the UK schedule...

2.7 DTaP vaccine does not contain thiomersal. The DTP vaccine used for babies at 2, 3 and 4 months (diphtheria, tetanus, wholecell pertussis vaccine – DTwP) does contain thiomersal. We do not intend to move presently to introduce DTaP vaccine for babies aged 2, 3 and 4 months, but this subject is kept under constant review. **(5)**

## Single dose immunisation

Because the mumps and rubella vaccines have never been delivered this way on a large scale, it isn't known if single dose presentation would be any safer than the triple dose (MMR). But the main problem with the single dose approach is that a certain amount of time has to pass between doses, leaving the child vulnerable to infection. Since immunisation rates began to fall (thanks to the MMR scare) there have been small outbreaks of measles here and there. It's certain that, if all parents chose the single dose option, there would be more cases of infection (in fact the first death from measles in the UK in over a decade was reported in April 2006).

In deciding whether to go ahead with the MMR jab for your child, you need to weigh up the risks. This means you need to know the risks associated with the illnesses your child may be susceptible to if it hasn't been inoculated.

## Measles

Measles is the most serious of the diseases the MMR vaccine is designed to protect us against, and one in which there's currently an upward trend in reported cases. Here are a few facts:

| Complications of Measles | R.isk |
| --- | --- |
| Diarrhoea | 1 in 6 |
| Ear infections | 1 in 20 |
| Pneumonia/bronchitis | 1 in 25 |
| Convulsions | 1 in 200 |
| Meningitis/encephalitis | 1 in 1000 |
| Death | 1 in 2500 – 5000 |
| Severe brain complications | 1 in 8000 |

The brain complications (subacute sclerosing panencephalitis) occur some years later in children who were under 2 years old when they caught measles.

And if you were wondering what the risks are of certain measles conditions with and without the MMR vaccine, here they are (though note these figures only include 1 dose of MMR):

| Complications | Risk after Natural Disease | Risk after 1st Dose MMR |
| --- | --- | --- |
| Convulsions | 1 in 200 | 1 in 1000 |
| Meningitis/encephalitis | 1 in 200 - 1 in 5000 | 1 in 1,000,000 |
| Blood clotting conditions | 1 in 3000 | 1 in 24,000 |
| Anaphylaxis | – | 1 in 100,000 |
| Deaths | 1 in 8000 –1 in 10,000 | 0 |

The wide variation in deaths range is due to age at death.

## Mumps

| Complications of mumps | Risk |
|---|---|
| Swollen testicles | 1 in 5 older males |
| Deafness | 1 in 25 |
| Pancreatitis | 1 in 30 |
| Meningitis/encephalitis | 1 in 200 –1 in 5,000 |

Deafness may improve with time but is usually permanent.

## Rubella

Here are the figures for rubella (German measles), which is dangerous because of the effects on the foetus if a pregnant woman catches it:

| Complications of rubella | Risk |
|---|---|
| Damage to foetus (multiple defects) | 9 in 10 pregnancies (1st 8-10 weeks) |
| Damage to foetus | 1 in 5-10 (10-16 weeks) |
| Bleeding disorders | 1 in 3,000 |
| Encephalitis | 1 in 6,000 |

## Egg allergy

The MMR vaccine is made using egg, and some people are concerned that if their child has an allergy to eggs it could be put at risk. If the allergic reaction is severe, ie resulting in breathing problems, swollen mouth and/or throat, and a rash, it's recommended that you tell your doctor or practice nurse so they can make alternative arrangements – which usually means a stay in the paediatric ward of your local hospital. There is increasing evidence that children with an allergy to eggs can be safely immunised without any problems.

## References against MMR

**http://members.jorsm.com**
Follow links to autism research monographs of Teresa Binstock. A lot of scientific data on the possible causes of autism including genetics, infection and mercury.

**http://www.nccn.net/~wwithin/mmr.htm**
Site dedicated to MMR information.

**http://www.nccn.net/~wwithin/MMR_VaccineTHROWER.pdf**
MMR vaccine, thimerosal and regressive or late onset autism (autistic enterocolitis). A review of the evidence for a link between vaccination and regressive autism. By David Thrower, parent of affected child.

**1** Lancet, 1998 Feb 28;351(9103):637-41
Ileal-lymphoid-nodular hyperplasia, non-specific colitis, and pervasive developmental disorder in children.
Wakefield AJ, Murch SH, Anthony A, Linnell J, Casson DM, Malik M, Berelowitz M, Dhillon AP, Thomson MA, Harvey P, Valentine A, Davies SE, Walker-Smith JA.
Inflammatory Bowel Disease Study Group, University Department of Medicine, Royal Free Hospital and School of Medicine, London, UK.

2: Digestive Diseases and Sciences 2001 Mar;46(3):658-60
Detection and sequencing of measles virus from peripheral mononuclear cells from patients with inflammatory bowel disease and autism.
Kawashima H, Mori T, Kashiwagi Y, Takekuma K, Hoshika A, Wakefield A.
Department of Paediatrics, Tokyo Medical University, Japan.

**3** Journal of Biomedical Science 2002 Jul-Aug;9(4):359-64
Abnormal measles-mumps-rubella antibodies and CNS autoimmunity in children with autism.
Singh VK, Lin SX, Newell E, Nelson C.
Department of Biology and Biotechnology Center, Utah State University, USA

## References in favour of MMR

**http://www.jr2.ox.ac.uk/bandolier/index.html**
**http://www.medinfo.co.uk**
Very useful factual site written by a medical doctor

**http://www.mmrthefacts.nhs.uk/**
NHS MMR info site

**http://www.who.int**
World Health Organisation

**http://www.nacc.org.uk**
National Organisation for Colitis and Crohn's

**4** American Journal of Human Genetics: online August 3rd 2005
Complex Gene Interactions Account for Autism Risk. Duke Center for Human
Genetics, Duke University Medical Center.
John Hussman, Ph.D, Michael Cuccaro, Ph.D
Collaborators: D.Q. Ma, P.L. Whithead, M.M. Menold, E.R. Martin, A.E. Ashley-
Koch, G.R. DeLong and J.R. Gilbert, all of Duke; H. Mei of North Carolina State
University; M.D. Ritchie of Vanderbilt University; and H.H. Wright, Ruth
Abramson of University of South Carolina.

**5 http://www.dh.gov.uk/assetRoot/04/01/36/40/04013640.pdf**
PL CPHO (2001)5: Current vaccine and immunisation issues
15 Oct 2001, letter from chief medical officer, chief nursing officer, chief pharma-
ceutical officer (Professor Liam Donaldson MSc, MD, FRCS(Ed), FRCP, FFPHM,
Sarah Mullally RN, MSc, BSc, Dr Jim Smith BPharm, PhD, FRPharmS, MCPP,
MIInfSci). Richmond House, 79 Whitehall, London SW1A 2NS

# 26 Other vaccines and the new 5x

In Autumn 2004 a new 5 in 1 vaccine replaced previous separate vaccines that covered polio, diphtheria, tetanus, pertussis (whooping cough) and Haemophilus influenza type B (Hib).

The polio vaccine was previously given orally and contained live virus, so was potentially capable of causing disease itself; this has been replaced with a dead version which is harmless (the UK is one of the last western countries to stop using oral polio). The part of the vaccine that contains pertussis has also been changed in order to cause fewer adverse reactions.

## Polio

Poliomyelitis is highly infectious and can cause paralysis if it reaches the central nervous system. The illness itself lasts about 2 weeks, though the complications can occasionally be fatal, but paralysis is lifelong, and more likely to affect adults and pregnant women. But the last case of natural polio infection in the UK was in 1982, and the last imported case in 1993.

## Diphtheria

This, as well as having an annoying second 'h' in it, is a nasty illness that can cause long term heart disease. Patients often need to go on ventilators to breathe, and it can be fatal. Immunisation was introduced nationally in 1940, leading to a huge fall in recorded cases. From 1986-2002, 103 cases of diphtheria were identified, and there were 2 deaths.

## Tetanus

Aka lockjaw, this affects the muscles and central nervous system, and can cause breathing problems. Because the tetanus bacterium is in soil and manure, any open cut has the potential to become infected – even if you live in the city (lovely organic veggies). Immunisation was begun nationally in 1961, and by the 70s tetanus had almost disappeared in children aged 5-15. In children younger than this there were no reported cases at all. In the UK there have been no cases of tetanus in newborns for over 30 years, and an average of just 6 cases a year in the rest of the population.

## Pertussis

Whooping cough can last for up to 10 weeks, causing long bouts of coughing and choking. Not such a problem for older kids and adults, in small babies it can be fatal, killing 1 in 500. Complications include collapsed lung and pneumonia, convulsions, brain damage, and repeated vomiting. Immunisation was introduced in the 1950s, causing a dramatic fall in cases, but there was a re-emergence in the 70s following a scare about the safety of the vaccine. Since 1992 there has been no fall in the number of cases in young babies – most patients admitted to hospital are below 6 months old. Because babies this young can't be immunised, the argument is that it's important to maintain 'herd immunity' so that the general level of risk is minimised.

## Haemophilus influenza Type B

Or Hib, to its enemies. It causes meningitis, septicaemia (blood poisoning) and epiglottitis (swelling of the epiglottis, which is the flap that covers your windpipe). Around 1 in 20 children who develop Hib meningitis die, and complications include brain damage, hearing and visual disorders, disability, delayed development and seizures. Epiglottitis can cause airway blockage that can be fatal, septic arthritis, osteomyelitis, cellulitis (a bacterial skin infection), pneumonia and pericarditis (swelling of the membrane around the heart).

Before vaccination began, children under 4 were most at risk, and more than $2/3$ of cases occurred in children under 2, with babies below 10–11 months being most vulnerable. 1 in 600 children developed some form of Hib by the time they were 5, and it was the most common cause of bacterial meningitis in juveniles. Every year in England and Wales, around 30 children died, and 80 were left with permanent brain damage and/or deafness.

After Hib immunisation began in 1992, cases of the disease in children under 5 dropped by 98%. In 2003 a booster campaign was initiated with call back of children between 6 months and 4 years.

## Latest developments

A press release published on 8th February 2006 and titled "Department of Health information on new vaccine for meningitis and septicaemia" concerned a pneumococcal vaccine added to the childhood immunisation programme to increase protection against meningitis and septicaemia. Invasive pneumococcal disease can cause these and pneumonia. Around 5000 cases occur in England and Wales every year, of which around 530 are in children under 2 years old. As many as 50 of these die.

In the USA a similar programme has had excellent results, with cases of the disease in young children dropping by 94%.

Routine pneumococcal vaccine is being introduced as part of a series of changes to the childhood immunisation programme. Other changes include retiming the present 3 doses of Meningitis C vaccine at 3 and 4 months, with a booster at 12 months. A booster of Hib will now be given at 12 months. The adjusted schedule looks like this:

- 2 months DTaP/IPV/Hib + pneumococcal vaccine
- 3 months DTaP/IPV/Hib + MenC vaccine
- 4 months DTaP/IPV/Hib + MenC + pneumococcal vaccine
- 12 months Hib/Men C
- 13 months MMR + pneumococcal vaccine

DTaP/IPV/Hib is a single vaccine that protects against diphtheria, tetanus, pertussis, polio and Hib. MenC protects against meningitis C, and Hib/ MenC is a combined vaccine protecting against Hib and Meningitis C.

The new vaccines are being introduced in 2006/07, and parents will be able to access information about the changes to the routine programme on the immunisation website (see link at the end of the chapter). **(1)**

The pneumococcal vaccine used for children aged 2 months to 5 years is pneumococcal conjugate vaccine, containing 7 capsular types of the disease. These are estimated to cause around 66% of all pneumococcal diseases, and 82% of those in children under 5 years.

The new 5 in 1 vaccine does not contain thiomersal, as the old vaccine did, and it's been used in Canada for 7 years. Is it controversial? You betcha. The preservative that replaced thiomersal (or thimerosal) in the Canadian vaccine (Pediarix) is 2-phenoxyethanol (2-PE), a main ingredient in antifreeze. Each dose of Pediarix contains 2.5mg of it, along with </= (less or equal to) 100mcg formaldehyde, </= 5% yeast protein, 4.5mg salt, and 0.85mg aluminium, among other things. 2-PE has been tested on rats and rabbits.

Pediarix has a higher rate of fever within the first 4 days compared to separately administered vaccines, but 98% of these resolve within that period.

## Useful websites/references

http://www.dh.gov.uk
http://www.immunisation.nhs.uk
http://www.drugs.com
Chemical components, what's in them, side effects etc

http://www.vran.org
Vaccination risk awareness network

## Other references

1   Dept of Health info on new vaccine for meningitis and septicaemia.
    Pneumococcal vaccine added to the childhood immunisation programme;
    more protection against meningitis and septicaemia
    Published:
    Wednesday 8 February 2006
    Reference number:
    2006/0056

# Part 5
# Feeding

## 27  Breastfeeding

Breast milk provides all the necessary nutrients (around 400 different ones) your baby needs, is hygienic and fresh, helps you bond, and there's no washing up. Breast milk is a complete food, containing hormones and antibodies necessary to your baby's health, and essential fatty acids (EFAs) that help with brain development. It changes as your baby grows, ensuring that it gets just what it needs.

### Weight control

One advantage is that breastfeeding helps you to use the fat you may have stored up during pregnancy (up to 0.5kg a month). The Department of Health recommends that you have an extra 450 calories of starchy carbohydrates a day during the 1st month in order to keep up with the demands made on your body. In the 2nd month this goes up to 530, and then 570 in the 3rd month. Other authorities think this may be too high, and instead recommend an extra intake of 300-400 calories daily for the first 3 months.

### Alcohol

Alcohol is not recommended. It does get into breast milk, and this can slow down your baby's progress in motor skills. Crawling and walking can be delayed. It may also make your baby restless and fractious, and as it can alter the smell of your milk, it could put the baby off feeding. High alcohol intake can also interfere with ejection of milk from the breast. Recommendations for alcohol consumption while breastfeeding state a maximum of 8 units a week, and no more than 2 units a day.

Alcohol is reckoned to clear the mother's bloodstream at a rate of one unit every two hours, so a wait of two hours per unit is recommended before breastfeeding the baby.

## Caffeine

Caffeine can make babies irritable ("Bloody hell woman, I hate pink") so you may find you need to lay off the coffee, tea, chocolate and cola drinks. It's recommended that you don't consume more than 300mg of caffeine a day:

- A mug of instant or brewed coffee contains 100mg
- A cup of coffee 75mg
- Cup of tea 50mg
- Can of cola up to 40mg
- Can of energy drink up to 80mg
- A 50g bar of chocolate up to 500mg

## Safe foods

It's now considered safe for you to eat foods that you may have been avoiding while pregnant, such as soft cheeses, eggs, tuna etc. This is because your baby is no longer in contact with your blood supply. And your immune system, which was lower during pregnancy, will now be functioning normally. But everything you consume will pass into your milk, and there are some foods that your baby just won't like ("Mother! Not foie gras with pop tarts, *please*"). Common triggers for colic include broccoli, cabbage, Brussels sprouts, and onion and dairy products.

## Smoking

The same provisos for smoking while pregnant apply to breast-feeding. Nicotine does get into breast milk, and it can decrease milk supply and cause nausea and vomiting in your baby. Bear in mind that this doesn't just mean smoking: patches and gum count too. Inhaling smoke increases your baby's chances of getting chest infections and otitis media (infection of the middle ear, or glue ear: risk is higher by 38-48%) and puts it at greater risk of SIDS (sudden infant death syndrome). If either you or your partner smokes, it is strongly recommended that you never do so in the baby's room, or anywhere near it.

## Medication

If you need to take any medication when breastfeeding, it's a good idea to ask your doctor or pharmacist if it's safe. Small amounts of many medications do get into breast milk, but most are harmless to the baby. If you are on anti-depressants, see Chapter 6 on Medication, which looks at how drugs affect babies via breastmilk. A Danish study done in 2006 examined current scientific data on whether mood stabilising drugs passed into breast milk, and if they did, what effect this had on the baby. The researchers didn't find much information, as very few studies have been done on this subject. But they do suggest that if a mother starts medication after the baby's birth (for post natal depression, say), it might be sensible to steer clear of fluoxetine and citalopram. If the mother is on lithium, breastfeeding should be avoided. The study concludes that premature, ill or chromosomally abnormal babies may be especially vulnerable to such drug exposure. [1]

Another 2006 study, reported in the British Journal of Pharmacology, looked at mothers who were using fluoxetine in the 3rd trimester and while breastfeeding. In 2 day old babies who had been exposed to the drug in the uterus, the concentrations of fluoxetine were the same as in the cord blood at birth. It took 2 months for these concentrations to fall away. Because newborns may have a decreased metabolism, this may lead to increased expo-sure. **(2)**

If you need anti-depressant treatment but are worried about drugs, you could do worse than try St John's Wort. A small but interesting study of 5 women who were taking St John's Wort while breast-feeding showed that, although the active ingredient (hyperforin) was excreted into breast milk at low levels, no side effects were seen in either mums or babies. **(3)**

## Health and development

What benefits does breastfeeding confer on your baby? Breast milk is a total food designed by nature to enable your baby to thrive. A variety of scientific studies have shown that breast fed babies grow better, get smarter, grow up healthier, are less likely to become obese, have fewer illnesses, sleep better, bond more closely with their mum, and are less likely to suffer from food allergies and gas-trointestinal problems. Their poo isn't so stinky either.

One of the most obvious benefits is the emotional closeness that grows between you and your baby. A study done in Nepal involv-ing 92 breastfeeding mothers wanted to find out how long they continued to breastfeed exclusively. Early skin-to-skin contact had a powerful influence on duration of breastfeeding up to 4-6 months, and was more important than how early the feeding start-ed. This included both vaginal and Caesarean births, and led the team to recommend that skin-to-skin contact plus early initiation of breastfeeding would be A Good Thing. **(4)**

## Wellbeing

An article published in Srpski Archiv za Celokupno Lekarstro, 2005 (what do you mean, you don't read Serbian?) investigated the importance of 2 enzymes: superoxide dismutase (SOD) and glu-tathione peroxidase (GSH-Px) in the antioxidant defence of new-born babies. The activity of these 2 enzymes in breast milk and colostrum was analysed, and also in the infants' gastric fluid and plasma. 63 mothers took part, and 45 babies in 4 groups: 10 breast-fed, 15 formula fed, 10 healthy breastfed newborns and 10 formula fed newborns with signs of neonatal sepsis. Activity of SOD was significantly lower in the gastric fluid of the formula fed babies than in that of the breastfed ones. It was however higher in the fluid of the babies with sepsis, indicating that it was taking part in combating the infection. The study concluded that the activities of both enzymes were important for adequate antioxidant defence in newborn babies, and that breastfeeding enables this. **(5)**

A Bristol, UK study of Australian 14 year olds looked at the circumstances of their early lives to try and determine what connections there might be between those and the children's intelligence. It found that the strongest indicators were family income, parental education and breastfeeding, which together explained 7.5% of the variation in intelligence. **(6)**

In Mexico (we're getting around, aren't we) researchers studied a group of 400 children, 200 of whom had been diagnosed with acute appendicitis; the other half hadn't. They wanted to know if breastfeeding had any effect on the later incidence of illness. They found that where the child had been exclusively breastfed, and especially for over 6 months, the risk of appendicitis was lower. **(7)**

Spain next: this time to see if breastfed babies settle into a good sleep/wake cycle as compared to bottle fed ones. Guess what? They do. 16 babies at 12 weeks old were divided into 2 groups (not a very big study but it's not the only one to reach this conclusion). One group was breastfed, the other not. Nocturnal sleep was increased in the breastfed babies, due to the tryptophan in the breast milk which acts as a regulator. **(8)**

Right, next stop New Zealand – don't say I never take you anywhere. Scientists at the Department of Paediatrics, University of Auckland investigated whether breastfeeding in infancy had an effect on intelligence at age 3.5 years. 550 children who took part in the Auckland Birthweight Collaborative Study were assessed.

About half of them were small for gestational age (SGA). Breastfeeding wasn't significantly related to intelligence scores in the total sample, despite a trend for longer periods of breastfeeding to be associated with higher scores. In the SGA group though, breastfeeding was significantly related to IQ. Those who were breastfed for longer than 12 months scored 6 points higher than non breastfed children. **(9)**

## Breastfeeding and asthma

There's some confusion over what effect breastfeeding has on respiratory problems such as asthma. While most authorities feel that it's beneficial, some studies have shown that it can apparently make things worse. Research done in 2002 and also reported by the University of Sheffield (as above) looked at 1037 children born in New Zealand between April 1972 and March 1973. They were assessed every 2-5 years from 9-26 years. 504 (49%) were breastfed and 533 (51%) were not. The breastfed children were more prone to atopy (allergies) such as dust mites, cats, and grass pollen, and also reported more prevalence of asthma. The study was adjusted for socioeconomic status, whether parents smoked, and parental history of allergy or asthma. The conclusion was that breastfeeding not only didn't have any protective effects, it may even increase the risk. **(10)**

A more recent piece of research reported in Pediatrics February 2006 sought to clarify this problem. It looked at the difference in exclusive breastfeeding results when done for 4 months, or 6 (as recommended by the American Academy of Pediatrics) on the risk of respiratory infection. Using data from the National Health and Nutrition Examination Survey III, a nationally representative cross-sectional home survey conducted from 1988 to 1994, 2277 children aged 6-24 months were included. The study found that when children were breastfed for 4 or up to 6 months, they had a higher risk of respiratory infection, but when they were breastfed for 6 months or more, the risk was reduced. **(11)**

And another study, reported in Journal of Allergy and Clinical Immunology March 2006 examined the hypothesis that it could be the early signs of problems such as atopic disease (see below) that caused the mothers to prolong breastfeeding, rather than the feeding causing the problem. 620 babies from Melbourne, Australia were involved. Results: 52 babies (8.4%) didn't establish breastfeeding, and 103 (25%) didn't establish exclusive breastfeeding (ie breast milk and nothing else). Early signs of atopic disease were associated with an approximately 28% reduction in risk of stopping exclusive breastfeeding. But there was no evidence of a relationship with risk of stopping breastfeeding completely. Their conclusion: that early signs of atopic disease might prolong the duration of exclusive breastfeeding, and this could mask a protective effect or even result in breastfeeding appearing to be a risk factor for the development of atopic disease. **(12)**

"Atopic" refers to a group of diseases where there is often an inherited tendency to develop other allergic conditions, such as asthma and hay fever.

Many health professionals feel that, whatever the possible risk regarding respiratory infection, the other advantages of breastfeeding far outweigh it.

A 1999 study from the University of Turku, Finland, looked at 100 babies who had atopic eczema. A strict elimination diet on the part of the mothers excluding trigger foods showed some improvements in the babies, but a greater improvement still came when breastfeeding ceased altogether. This was not interpreted as a recommendation not to breastfeed, because the incidence of atopic eczema is far higher in bottle fed babies. But it is clear that allergens in the mothers' milk were the trigger for the eczema in the babies, and the elimination diet did help. Only when the reaction is extreme or the baby has impaired growth should breastfeeding be stopped. **(13)**

The best way of avoiding allergic reactions in a newborn baby, if you have a family history of allergies on both sides, is to exclusively breastfeed (ie no formula, water etc) for a minimum of 6 months (one note of caution here: this can lead to vitamin D deficiency, as breast milk is often low in this vitamin, so you may need to take a supplement). And keep your diet free of known triggers like nuts, dairy produce and eggs. And fish. Plus alcohol, caffeine, soya, broccoli, cabbage, onions (in case of colic) and no fags. Like the man said "I may not actually be living longer, but it sure as hell feels like it." Still, look on the bright side: you'll be getting so little sleep that you won't notice the first 3 years.

## Other references

1   CNS Drugs 2006;20(3):187-98
    Use of Psychotropic Medications in Treating Mood Disorders during Lactation :
    Practical Recommendations.
    Eberhard-Gran M, Eskild A, Opjordsmoen S.
    Division of Epidemiology, Norwegian Institute of Public Health, Oslo, Norway.

2   British Journal of Clinical Pharmacology
    Stereoselective disposition of fluoxetine and norfluoxetine during pregnancy
    and breast-feeding.
    Kim J, Riggs KW, Misri S, Kent N, Oberlander TF, Grunau RE, Fitzgerald C, Rurak
    DW.
    Department of Psychiatry, University of British Columbia.

3   Journal of Clinical Psychiatry
    St. John's wort (Hypericum perforatum) and breastfeeding: plasma and breast
    milk concentrations of hyperforin for 5 mothers and 2 infants.
    Klier CM, Schmid-Siegel B, Schafer MR, Lenz G, Saria A, Lee A, Zernig G.
    Department of Child and Adolescent Neuropsychiatry, Medical University
    Vienna, Vienna, Austria, and the Division of Clinical Pharmacology and
    Toxicology, Hospital for Sick Children, Toronto, Ontario, Canada

4   Nepal Medical College Journal
    Effect of early mother-baby close contact over the duration of exclusive breast-
    feeding.
    Vaidya K, Sharma A, Dhungel S.
    Department of Pediatrics, Nepal Medical College, Jorpati, Kathmandu.

5   Srpski Arhiv za Celokupno Lekarstro 2005 Dec;133 Suppl2:108-12
    Importance of breast-feeding in antioxidant defence

Article in Serbian
No authors listed

**6** Paediatric and Perinatal Epidemiology 2006 Mar;20(2):148-62
Early life predictors of childhood intelligence: findings from the Mater-University study of pregnancy and its outcomes.
Lawlor DA, Najman JM, Batty GD, O'Callaghan MJ, Williams GM, Bor W.
Department of Social Medicine, University of Bristol, Bristol, UK

**7** Gaceta Medica de Mexico
Early breastfeeding as a risk factor for acute appendicitis in children
Article in Spanish
Gomez-Alcala AV, Hurtado-Guzman A.
Coordinacion de Investigacion en Salud, Delegacion Sonora, IMSS, Mexico

**8** Neuro Endocrinology Letters
The circadian rhythm of tryptophan in breast milk affects the rhythms of 6-sulfatoxymelatonin and sleep in newborns.
Cubero J, Valero V, Sanchez J, Rivero M, Parvez H, Rodriguez AB, Barriga C.
Department of Physiology, Faculty of Science, Extremadura University, Badajoz, Spain

**9** Acta Paediatrica 2005 Jul;94(7):827-9
Breastfeeding and intelligence of preschool children.
Slykerman RF, Thompson JM, Becroft DM, Robinson E, Pryor JE, Clark PM, Wild CJ, Mitchell EA.
Department of Paediatrics, University of Auckland, Auckland, New Zealand.

**10** 03270. Lancet 2002; 360:901
Long-term Relation Between Breastfeeding and Development of Atopy and Asthma in Children and Young Adults: a Longitudinal Study.
M Sears, J Greene, A Willan, D Taylor, E Flannery, J Cowan, G Herbison, R Poulton

**11** Pediatrics 2006 Feb;117(2):425-32
Full breastfeeding duration and associated decrease in respiratory tract infection in US children.
Chantry CJ, Howard CR, Auinger P.
Department of Pediatrics, University of California Davis Medical Center, Sacramento, USA

**12** Journal of Allergy and Clinical Immunology 2006 Mar;117(3):682-7 Epub
Atopic disease and breast-feeding—cause or consequence?
Lowe AJ, Carlin JB, Bennett CM, Abramson MJ, Hosking CS, Hill DJ, Dharmage SC.

Centre for Molecular, Environmental, Genetic and Analytic Epidemiology, The University of Melbourne, and the Department of Allergy, Royal Children's Hospital, Australia

**13** Journal of Pediatrics 1999 Jan;134(1):27-32
Isolauri E, Tahvanainen A, Peltola T, Arvola T
Department of Pediatrics, University of Turku, Finland.

# 28 Bottle feeding

All the above might make it sound like child abuse if you don't breastfeed all day every day (and night) for at least 6 months. But here we are in modern Britain and lots of mums have a career. It's difficult to be taken seriously in a meeting with a squalling infant under one arm. And as for whipping your boobs out – you could be CEO in 3 months.

There are other factors too: lack of milk, illness, fatigue, just not wanting to (this is allowed by the way), or being a dad. Thousands of babies are reared perfectly well and happily by bottle, so if this is your method by choice or necessity, just relax and enjoy it. One major advantage of bottle feeding is that you can both do it, which means bonding time for dad and rest time for mum. Granny, grandad and older siblings can have a go too, so it can involve the whole family if you want it to.

## Formula

Most formula baby milk is based on cows milk and uses whey protein, lactose and casein. Babies can be lactose intolerant, so a switch to a lactose free formula is then recommended. However, around 20% of babies have an allergic reaction to both. But if you don't have a family history of allergies, you should be fine with either. There are hydrolysed formulae, which use bovine casein or whey, but treat it to make it hypoallergenic. Sadly, these tend not to taste very nice apparently (I must admit I haven't tried them, as far as I can remember). Goat's milk formula is not approved for use in Europe, but apparently donkey milk is the closest in composition to that of humans. So you'll be all right if you live in Blackpool.

## Useful resources/references

**http://www.forparentsbyparents.com**
Good support website run by 2 parents, discussions, comments etc from parents about all sorts of issues.

**http://www.babycentre.co.uk**
Fantastic, comprehensive website that's scientific, informative and friendly

**www.babyworld.co.uk**
Chatty and informative site

**http://www.marchofdimes.com**
March of Dimes: big US site

# 29 Weaning

As far as allergies go, the official line is that you should delay the introduction of solid foods until your baby is six months old. By then it will be better adapted to cope with any allergens (foods that may cause an allergic reaction). For more on this see the next chapter. At six months, start with rice, lamb, non-citrus fruit and non-legume vegetables. Keep away from potential allergens altogether for the 1st year, and only introduce eggs, peanuts and bony fish after 2 or 3 years.

## When to wean?

A big question. Some mothers can't wait, and others are still at it several years down the line. In many cultures children are breast-fed for a couple of years, but this is often seen as impractical in the west. It's a matter of choice that's entirely up to you, but with prevailing opinion being somewhere along the lines of 'still breast-feeding at 18 months – how weird' it can be difficult to stick to your guns (this in a culture that uses women's breasts to sell everything from sun tan lotion to music, but which throws up its hands in horror if you breastfeed in the park).

The official line is that you breastfeed for as long as possible (within reason; bitty at 23 is a tad extreme) but start introducing solid food around 6 months. Your baby won't get enough iron from milk alone beyond this age. Before 4 months the baby's digestive system may not be ready to cope with it, and there's an increased risk of respiratory illness, allergic reaction or food sensitivity. However all babies are different, and if their baby is constantly hungry before this age, many parents do start feeding something bland like baby rice despite the official advice. Babies need to learn how to swallow solid material, so the first few spoonfuls may slither out of its mouth, but it will soon get the hang of it. Whether or not it likes the taste is another matter, and you may find your kitchen walls artexed with Finest Organic Babygoo.

# 30 Allergies

Does what you eat affect whether or not your baby has allergies? The short answer is yes. If it has a reaction to something you've eaten it may get a skin rash or hives, start wheezing, and produce green or slimy poo. Possibly all at once. However, breastfeeding in general prevents allergies.

The earlier a baby is exposed to allergenic foods, the more likely it is to have a reaction. Its digestive system isn't designed to cope with anything except mother's milk, and its immune system isn't finished yet. Your colostrum contains an antibody called secretory immunoglobulin A (sIgA), which coats the inside of your baby's gut to help it be resistant to allergens. Mature milk does this too. It's only around 6 weeks old that babies start to produce immunoglobulins (antibodies), and at about 6 months they start to make their own sIgA.

A true food allergy causes an immediate reaction after ingestion, seconds or minutes after swallowing. A food intolerance, on the other hand, generally has a more delayed reaction, often hours or even days later. It usually involves the digestive tract and not the immune system, and causes discomfort but is not life threatening.

Symptoms of a food allergy include itchy skin (hives or urticaria), swollen or itchy tongue and lips, sneezing, blocked or runny nose (rhinitis), wheezing, coughing and shortness of breath.

Anaphylaxis is the most severe form of allergic reaction and it requires emergency medical treatment. Symptoms are similar to those above, but more extreme, including tightening of the throat, difficulty breathing, and feeling faint. Skin may become pale and clammy. Anaphylaxis can lead to unconsciousness or death, so call 999 or take your baby to casualty immediately. It can be triggered by even minuscule amounts of the allergen, and in children the most common culprits are eggs, milk and nuts. Medication, bee or wasp stings, and latex can also bring on anaphylaxis.

For food intolerance, the symptoms are stomach pain or colic, bloating, wind, diarrhoea, and occasionally, vomiting.

Somewhere around 5-8% of children develop a food allergy, and 90% of them will grow out of it, although they may develop allergy related conditions like asthma, hayfever, eczema or rhinitis later on in life. Allergy usually appears in babies with feeding problems and a strong family background of allergy. If one parent has allergies, there's a 37% risk of the baby developing them, and if both parents do, this increases to 62%.

## Nuts

A study reported by the University of Sheffield Centre of Pregnancy Nutrition looked at whether peanut allergens could be detected in breast milk. 23 lactating women were given 50g of dry roasted peanuts to eat, after which their milk was sampled at hourly intervals. Peanut protein, including 2 major allergens, was detected in 11 of the 23 subjects' milk. In 10 of the 11 it showed up within 2 hours of ingestion. (1)

Experts recommend that if either of the baby's parents, or any close relatives or previous children, have a history of hayfever, asthma, eczema or other allergies, it's best to avoid eating peanuts and products that contain them while you're breastfeeding. The same applies to other nuts (although strictly speaking peanuts are not nuts but legumes). Chestnuts, on the other hand, rarely cause nut allergy, but if you're allergic to latex, you may well be allergic to chestnuts as well.

What about peanut oil? This is often used in cooking or salads, especially by commercial food preparers such as chip shops, restaurants and cafés. However, these will mostly be using refined peanut oil which has had the protein removed, and is not an allergen. But ... some people have nevertheless had a reaction to it. The problem may be that different refineries have different standards of thoroughness. Also the oil may have had something added to it. Unrefined or cold pressed peanut oil is a definite no-no if you're avoiding peanuts.

## Eggs

Interestingly, there is some evidence to suggest that babies delivered via Caesarean section are over 4 times more likely to develop an egg allergy than vaginally born babies. The reason seems to be that Caesarean section delays colonisation of the baby's gut with beneficial bacteria that help prevent allergies. Therefore it's a good idea to breastfeed a baby born this way. It's also possible that women who take probiotics through the 3rd trimester and during breastfeeding may help prevent their baby getting allergies.

It's usually egg white that babies are allergic to, rather than the yolk. This is because it's the white that has the protein in it. And because the protein molecules of eggs are quite large, and easily affected by heat, cooked eggs may not cause a problem. Thus small amounts of egg in pasta or cake, for example, may be safe for the mother to eat.

Egg allergy is most common in babies under 1 year old, which is why it's recommended that they aren't fed any egg in that time. Most children grow out of it.

## Dairy

There are more than 20 substances in cow's milk that have been shown to be human allergens, and the protein has been found to enter breast milk. This can sensitise a baby so that even tiny amounts of cow milk triggers an allergic response. Colic and vomiting are common reactions, as is eczema. Cow milk can also cause sleeplessness in small babies.

With regard to formula, some babies are reacting to the large amounts of cow milk they're being given. It's the equivalent of drinking around 8 litres a day – which might make anybody sick.

If you cut dairy products out of your diet, you need to make sure you and your baby get your calcium from somewhere else. Babies need 400mg a day, and you need 1200mg. Green leafy veggies are a good source, or you can take a supplement.

## Useful websites/references

1   03326. Detection of Peanut Allergens in Breast Milk of Lactating Women. JAMA 2001;285;1746-8
     P Vadas, Y Wai, W Burks, B Perelman

**http://www.allergy-clinic.co.uk**
Excellent allergy site

**http://www.allergy-network.co.uk**
Good solid information site

**http://www.maara.org**
Medical homepage of the Midlands Asthma and Allergy Research Association

# Glossary

| Word or term | Meaning or explanation |
|---|---|
| 2-Phenoxyethanol | Preservative used in vaccines |
| Abruptio placentae | Placenta partially detaches from uterine wall |
| Allergen | Substance that triggers allergic reaction |
| Amniotic bands etc | Structures found in amniotic fluid |
| Aneuploidy | Having less or more than the normal number of chromosomes |
| Apgar score | Five point scoring system to assess distress in newborns |
| Artificially rupturing the membrane | Using a probe to break membranes to induce birth |
| Blighted ovum | An egg has implanted, but not developed into an embryo |
| Caesarean section | Removal of baby via incision in abdomen |
| Carrier | If you have 1 mutated gene in a pair, thus do not have the disease but can pass it on |
| Cephalhaematoma | Blood blister that sometimes appears on baby's scalp after ventouse |
| Chromosomal abnormalities | Too many or too few chromosomes, or they are in the wrong order |
| Crown rump length | Method of measuring baby's length used in 1st trimester |
| Doula | Trained birth attendant |
| Down's syndrome | Chromosomal abnormality also called trisomy 21 |
| Epidemiology | The medical science that deals with the frequency, distribution and control of disease |
| Epidural | Painkilling injection into spine during labour |
| Episiotomy | Cut made in perineum between vagina and anus |

| | |
|---|---|
| Etiologic significance | A causative factor |
| Febrile seizures | Fever induced convulsions in babies and small children |
| FISH | Fluorescence in-situ hybridisation, or rapid aneuploidy testing |
| Forceps | Pair of large, curved tongs used to assist delivery |
| Gastroschisis | Imperfect closure of baby's abdomen |
| IgE | Immunoglobulin E, antibody triggered by allergies |
| IUGR | Intra Uterine Growth Retardation |
| Karyotyping | Chromosome analysis, genetic testing |
| Membrane sweep | Membranes surrounding the baby are separated from cervix to induce labour |
| Meptid | Analgesic used during labour |
| Missed miscarriage | Embryo which began to develop then stopped, and remains in the uterus |
| Naegele's rule | A way of calculating due date |
| Narcan | Drug injected into baby to reverse adverse effects of pethidin |
| Neural tube defects | Tube surrounding central nervous system doesn't close up properly ie spina bifida |
| Neurogenesis | Nerve growth |
| Norepinephrine | Hormone |
| Oedema | Fluid retention causing swelling, usually in lower leg |
| Oxytocin | Hormone |
| PCA | Patient controlled analgesia |
| Pelvic floor muscles (Kegel) | Muscular sling that, when weakened, can cause incontinence |
| Perinatal | Before birth |
| Pertussis | Whooping cough |
| Pethidine | Analgesic and anti spasmodic |

# Glossary

| | |
|---|---|
| Phenotype | Outward physical manifestation |
| Placebo | Dummy pill used in blind testing |
| Placenta praevia | Placenta planted low in uterus, causing obstruction |
| Prostaglandin | Hormone like substance that triggers contractions |
| Retroplacental or chorionic haematoma | Blood clots under the placenta |
| SIDS | Sudden infant death syndrome |
| Spina bifida | Neural tube defect |
| SUA | Single umbilical artery |
| Syntocinon | Synthetic form of oxytocin |
| Talipes Equinovarus | Rocker bottom feet |
| Teratogenic | Causing harm to foetus within 1st trimester |
| Thiomersal/Thimerosal | Preservative used in some vaccines |
| Transient PNA | Temporary poor neonatal adaptation |
| Trisomy 21 | Chromosomal abnormality: Down's syndrome |
| Ultrasound markers | Physical signs seen via ultrasound that may or may not indicate abnormality |
| Vaginal scan | Ultrasound scan done via vaginal probe |
| VBAC | Vaginal birth after Caesarean |
| Venepuncture | Needle inserted into a vein |
| Ventouse | Vacuum suction used to assist delivery |
| VKDB | Vitamin K deficiency bleeding |

# Contact us

You're welcome to contact White Ladder Press if you have any questions or comments for either us or the authors. Please use whichever of the following routes suits you.

**Phone:** 01803 813343 between 9am and 5.30pm

**Email:** enquiries@whiteladderpress.com

**Fax:** 01803 813928

**Address:** White Ladder Press, Great Ambrook, Near Ipplepen, Devon TQ12 5UL

**Website: www.whiteladderpress.com**


# What can our website do for you?

If you want more information about any of our books, you'll find it at **www.whiteladderpress.com**. In particular you'll find extracts from each of our books, and reviews of those that are already published. We also run special offers on future titles if you order online before publication. And you can request a copy of our free catalogue.

Many of our books have links pages, useful addresses and so on relevant to the subject of the book. You'll also find out a bit more about us and, if you're a writer yourself, you'll find our submission guidelines for authors. So please check us out and let us know if you have any comments, questions or suggestions.

# Babies
## for Beginners
### Roni Jay

**"A perfect first book for all new mums and dads confused by parenthood."** *Pregnancy*

At last, here is the book for every new parent who's never been quite sure what a cradle cap is and whether you need one. *Babies for Beginners* cuts away the crap – the unnecessary equipment, the overfussy advice – and gives you the absolute basics of babycare: keep the baby alive, at all costs, and try to stop it getting too hungry.

From bedtime to bathtime, mealtime to playtime, this book highlights the core *objective* of each exercise (for example, get the baby bathed) and the *key focus* (don't drown it). By exploding the myths around each aspect of babycare, the book explains what is necessary and what is a bonus; what equipment is essential and what you can do without.

*Babies for Beginners* is the perfect book for every first time mother who's confused by all the advice and can't believe it's really necessary to spend that much money. And it's the ultimate guide for every father looking for an excuse to get out of ante-natal classes.

Roni Jay is a professional author whose books include *KIDS & Co: winning business tactics for every family*. She is the mother of three young children, and stepmother to three grown up ones.

*This edition contains new material*

£7.99

# From **Lad** to **Dad**

## How to survive as a pregnant father

"Stephen Giles describes the fears and frustrations of impending fatherhood with honesty and humour, along with practical help and advice." **Lawrence Dallaglio**

You've done it – she's pregnant. Now all you have to do is sit back, put your feet up and wait for the congratulations of friends and family. Right?

Wrong. Suddenly it's all about her and you're relegated to the sidelines, facing nine long months of getting lost in her ever expanding shadow.

So forget the laid back lifestyle (you'll be too busy waiting on her every whim). Forget late night socialising (she'll be too tired). And forget sex, obviously. At least in any form you'd recognise. Instead you've got to learn a whole new role, and fast.

Now at least you have one fellow traveller to take your side and give you the attention you deserve. Stephen Giles has charted his own journey from lad to dad and shares his ignorance, humiliations, frustrations, inadequacies and downright sodding terror. Along the way he guides you through the minefield of dismissive midwives, scary hospital visits, mood swings (hers as well as yours), and the looming prospect of having to reinvent yourself as a halfway decent dad.

He also passes on the answers to many of his own questions, along with a mass of practical and realistic advice, and reassures you that if he can survive as a pregnant father, so can you. In fact not only can you survive, but you can emerge at the end of it all feeling bloody fantastic.

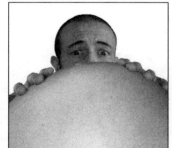

**"Here is the proof that you are not alone. Nor are you useless, powerless or redundant. You're the daddy, almost. And absolutely nothing beats that."**

**£7.99**

# You're the **Daddy**

## From nappy mess to happiness in one year
## The art of being a great dad

## Stephen **Giles**

And you thought pregnancy was a steep learning curve? Once the baby is born, your life turns upside down. Sure, a lot of the changes are great, but they're all new and you set out with barely a clue how to cope. Life is packed with new challenges to face and new skills to learn.

That's why you need a friend and guide to reassure you and hold your hand through that crucial first year.

A follow-up to his popular and highly entertaining *From Lad to Dad How to survive as a pregnant father*, Stephen Giles now sets out his progress through the first year of his baby's life. Once again he tells his story in journal form with great humour, and plenty of practical ideas and advice for other first time fathers on topics such as:

- the conflict between work pressure and sleepless nights
- division of labour at home
- being the breadwinner, the main carer or any combination of the two
- your changing relationship with your partner
- keeping 'competitive dad syndrome' under control

Stephen will help you ensure that by the end of your first year not only will you be able to change a nappy in your sleep (should you be lucky enough to get any) but, more importantly, you'll have mastered the art of being a great dad.

**£7.99**

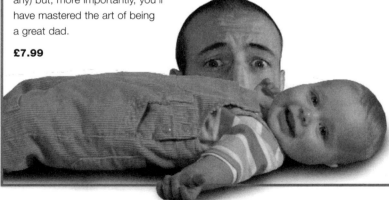

# Index

# Index